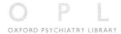

OXFORD PSYCHIATRY LIBRARY

Bipolar Disorder

O P L

OXFORD PSYCHIATRY LIBRARY

Bipolar Disorder

Lakshmi N Yatham

Professor of Psychiatry
Vice Chair for Research and International Affairs
Department of Psychiatry
The University of British Columbia
Vancouver, British Columbia
Canada

Gin S Malhi

Professor and Head
Discipline of Psychiatry
Sydney Medical School, University of Sydney
Director, CADE Clinic
Royal North Shore Hospital
Sydney, Australia

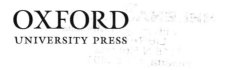

OXFORD

UNIVERSITY PRESS

*This book has been printed digitally and produced in a standard specification
in order to ensure its continuing availability*

OXFORD
UNIVERSITY PRESS

Great Clarendon Street, Oxford OX2 6DP
United Kingdom

Oxford University Press is a department of the University of Oxford.
It furthers the University's objective of excellence in research, scholarship,
and education by publishing worldwide. Oxford is a registered trade mark of
Oxford University Press in the UK and in certain other countries

First published 2011
Reprinted 2013

British Library Cataloguing in Publication Data
Data available

Library of Congress Cataloging in Publication Data
Data available

ISBN 978-0-19-956230-5

Contents

Preface

Bipolar disorder is common, has complex presentations, and causes significant morbidity and mortality. Not surprisingly then, a vast amount of research has been conducted particularly over the past two decades to understand the clinical complexity, course, causes and treatment of this condition. For an average clinician or health care professional providing care for patients with bipolar disorder, it is a daunting task to keep abreast of these advances and more importantly make sense of what is clinically relevant.

The purpose of this book then is to provide a concise summary of information that is pertinent for a clinician managing patients. The evolution of the concept of bipolar disorder is provided before describing the modern concept of diagnostic sub-types, clinical features, and tips for clinicians for diagnosis and differential diagnosis of this condition. This succinct overview of terminology and definitions is important as it provides an understanding of the language used in the management of bipolar disorder. The chapter on neurobiology is deliberately kept simple and brief to give a flavour in terms of the progress that has been achieved to date. The chapters on pharmacotherapy and psychological treatments summarize the latest evidence while the chapters on treatment guidelines and special populations provide guidance for clinicians in making treatment choices. These chapters are key and provide practical recommendations that most clinicians should be able to incorporate into their management practices. The main message however, is that although pharmacotherapy is the cornerstone of management of bipolar disorder, adjunctive psychosocial treatments palpably improve functioning and outcome.

Ultimately, the optimal management of bipolar disorder includes a collaborative team approach that incorporates both pharmacological and psychological treatments. Pivotal in this is the therapeutic alliance between patients with the illness and their treating clinician. In this context, we hope that this book will become an important pocket resource for clinicians managing bipolar disorder in conjunction with their patients.

Lakshmi N. Yatham

Gin S. Malhi

Abbreviations

5-HT	5-hydroxytryptamine – serotonin
ACTH	Adrenocorticotropic hormone (corticotropin)
BDI	Beck Depression Inventory
BDNF	Brain-derived neurotrophic factor
CAD	Coronary artery disease
CANMAT	Canadian Network for Mood and Anxiety Treatments
DSM-IV-TR	Diagnostic and Statistical Manual of Mental Disorders, Fourth Edition, Third Revision
ECT	Electroconvulsive therapy
EPS	Extrapyramidal symptoms
HAMD	Hamilton Rating Scale for Depression
ICD-10	International Classification of Diseases (ICD-10)
LAI	Long-acting injection
MADRS	Montgomery-Asberg Depression Rating Scale
MAOI	Monoamine oxidase inhibitor
MDD	Major depressive disorder
NARI	Noradrenaline (norepinephrine) reuptake inhibitor
NaSSA	Noradrenergic and selective serotonin antagonists
NE	Norepinephrine
NIMH	National Institute of Mental Health
NSAIDs	Nonsteroidal anti-inflammatory drugs
rTMS	Repetitive transcranial magnetic stimulation
SERT	5-HT reuptake transporter
SGAs	Second-generation antipsychotics
TCA	Tricyclic antidepressant
TSH	Thyroid-stimulating hormone
VNS	Vagus nerve stimulation

Chapter 1

Introduction and historical context

Key points

- Bipolar disorder, formerly known as manic-depressive illness, is not a new illness
- Bipolar disorder emerges in the formative years of growth with significant impact on cognitive and emotional development
- There is no cure for bipolar disorder
- Treatment focus is early detection, control of symptoms and prophylaxis.

Disorders of mood are not new and descriptions of changes in emotion have been identified in both ancient Greek and Persian writings. Aretaeus of Cappadocia, a practitioner in Rome, recognized almost 2,000 years ago that depression and mania are in essence part of the 'human condition'. His early descriptions capture not only the nature of the various emotional states but also track the changes in mood that occur longitudinally. In his accounts he described individuals who at times were 'very sad and sorrowful', without obvious cause, and yet at other times these same individuals became 'excessively talkative' and 'overly confident' such that they 'danced throughout the night'. He was perhaps the first to meaningfully connect mania and depression and identify their cyclical nature as demonstrated by his comment 'it appears to me that melancholy is the commencement and a part of mania'. Remarkably, this astute early insight had little impact upon subsequent thinking. Indeed it is not until the 19th century when both Jean Pierre Falret (1794–1870) and Jules Baillarger (1809–1890) independently posit that a single illness could perhaps present with the separate faces of depression and mania that this concept surfaces once again. Falret described this as 'circular insanity' and along with Baillarger provided the necessary foundation, upon which Emil Kraepelin with his own meticulous observations of both depression and mania created a new entity namely, 'manic depressive insanity'. Interestingly, Kraepelin also drew upon the work of Ewald Hecker and Karl Ludwig Kahlbaum, so as to ultimately separate manic depression (unipolar or major depression and bipolar disorder) from dementia praecox (schizophrenia), a fundamental classificatory division that holds to this day.

It is important to note, however that the 'face' of manic depressive insanity has changed considerably over the past century. The majority of patients encountered by early psychiatrists and physicians dealing with the mentally ill were residents of asylums that were severely unwell. Most had psychotic symptoms in conjunction with depression and mania and the majority of early observations do not explicitly partition patients according to changes in mood per se. Further, bipolarity is a relatively recent concept that has emerged in the middle of the 20th century. However, a key distinction that Kraepelin did make between schizophrenia and the affective psychoses and one that is of significant clinical importance relates to the outcome of the respective illnesses. Specifically, he viewed schizophrenia as an illness that invariably has a poor outcome, with a progressive course, functional impairment and ongoing residual symptoms. In comparison, manic depression was regarded as being periodic (episodic) and with a potential for complete recovery. Interestingly, these observations and views upon which much of the current classification systems are predicated are now being revisited and challenged.

In the course of this book we will briefly examine the issues that surround detection and diagnosis of bipolar disorder and its classification. We will also consider how, with the advent of modern tests and technology, the identification of deficits and changes that may form the basis of neurobiological markers, alter our perspective and understanding of the illness.

Over the past decade there has been a growing interest in bipolar disorders that has been fuelled largely by the development of new treatments or new indications for existing medications. Equally exciting, and perhaps more important in the long term, has been the growing appreciation of psychological interventions and the importance of non-pharmacological measures. Despite advances in our understanding, with better treatments and greater insights into the illness there is still no cure for bipolar disorder and management is in effect symptomatic with an increasing focus on prophylaxis. Early detection, optimal pharmacological and psychological management that include episode control and prevention of further mood episodes likely lead to improved functioning and long term outcome. With better understanding, there has been broader acceptance of the illness at both personal and societal levels. However, as with all psychiatric disorders stigma remains a significant problem. Further, aspects of the illness are still confused with personality and wrongly associated with genius or conversely a lack of intelligence.

At the core of the illness is the individual. Bipolar disorder, as we will see, emerges at a formative time in life and impacts upon cognitive and emotional development and this leads to interpersonal, educational and financial difficulties that potentially have a life long impact. Beyond the individual, the illness also impacts upon the immediate family and friends of the person suffering, and thus produces a tremendous burden both for the person affected and the community as a whole. Individuals with bipolar disorder often experience this aspect of their illness and its consequences as an added burden that comprises guilt and shame. The focus of treatments has therefore embraced these issues and attempts to achieve longer term improvement, with interest in diminishing the impact of the illness and its treatments, on cognition and overall social and occupational functioning.

However, the majority of our present treatments remain imprecise either because of incomplete efficacy or side effects that limit tolerability. Whilst this remains the state of affairs, and in the absence of a cure, it is not surprising that individuals with bipolar disorder question the need for treatment. At the heart of their concern is the view that some treatments and interventions make them 'feel' different and take away an aspect of their personality. It is important therefore that we continue to strive for a better understanding of bipolar disorder so as to be able to develop targeted treatments that not only manage the acute episodes and treat their recurrence but hopefully treat the causes of the illness and ultimately achieve a cure.

References and further reading

Benazzi F (2007). Bipolar disorder-focus on bipolar II disorder and mixed depression. *The Lancet*, **369**, 935.

Ghaemi SN, Baldessarini RJ (2007). The manic-depressive spectrum and mood stabilization: Kraepelin's ghost. *Psychotherapy and Psychosomatics*, **76**, 65.

Kraeplin E (1921). *Manic-depressive insanity and paranoia*. Edinburgh: E&S Livingstone.

Mondimore FM (2005). Kraepelin and manic-depressive insanity: an historical perspective. *International Review of Psychiatry*, **17**, 49–52.

Chapter 2

Recognizing bipolar disorder: clinical features and diagnoses

Key points

- Although mania defines bipolar disorder, depressive episodes are more common in this condition
- All patients presenting with depressive symptoms must be screened for a diagnosis of bipolar disorder by routinely asking for symptoms of mania/hypomania
- Co-morbidity of substance and alcohol abuse and other psychiatric disorders is common in bipolar disorder
- A careful history, drug screen, physical examination and other investigations may be necessary to make an accurate and reliable diagnosis of bipolar disorder.

2.1 Clinical presentation

Classic bipolar disorder is a recurrent episodic illness that is usually cyclical in nature. It is characterized by episodes of hypomania or mania that distinguish it from unipolar (major) depression and these 'highs' are usually interspersed amongst episodes of bipolar depression that are commonly referred to as 'lows'. Diagnostically, the illness is further subdivided into bipolar I and bipolar II disorder on the basis of duration and severity of manic symptoms (see Table 2.1 and Figure 2.1 for details of the signs, symptoms and diagnostic classification). With time the classification of bipolar disorder has expanded to include additional subtypes such that it is increasingly viewed as a spectrum of illnesses. Nevertheless, of the many subtypes proposed, bipolar I and bipolar II, as defined in DSM IV, are the most widely accepted (see Figure 2.1).

Table 2.1 The signs and symptoms of bipolar disorder		
Sign/Symptom	Mania	Bipolar Depression
APPEARANCE	Colourful, strange, garish makeup or dress style	Disinterest in personal appearance, grooming and hygiene
MOOD	Prolonged elation/ euphoria Excessively optimistic or cheerful Heightened irritability	Feelings of sadness Suicidal ideation
SPEECH	Talking fast and loudly Difficult to interrupt	Speech is slowed Monosyllabic and monotonous
ACTIVITY	Risk-taking behavior Impulsive Increased psychomotor activity (restlessness)	Difficulty with initiating tasks Diminished interest in hobbies Decreased psychomotor activity
SLEEP	Decreased need for sleep	Early morning waking with insomnia OR Hypersomnia with daytime napping
COGNITION	Difficulties with planning, reasoning and decision-making Distractible	Reduced ability to concentrate Difficulties with memory
SELF PERCEPTION/ THINKING	Exaggerated self-confidence Grandiose thinking	Reduced self-esteem Feelings of worthlessness and guilt Pessimistic thoughts and sense of hopelessness

2.1.1 Signs and symptoms

2.1.1.1 *Manic episode*

Mania defines bipolar disorder and typically, it is an easily identified discrete change in mental state during which the individual is euphoric, expansive or irritable in terms of mood (See Box 2.1). In addition the person usually describes a decreased need for sleep, along with a marked increase in energy, and a strong desire to engage in risk-taking behaviour. Often attention is limited and the person is distractible. Further, individuals commonly describe their thoughts as 'racing' which manifests as talking much faster than usual, and it is often difficult for health care professionals to interrupt the patient. Their judgment is

Box 2.1 DSM-IV criteria for mania

1. A distinct period of abnormally and persistently elevated, expansive or irritable mood, lasting at least one week (or any duration if hospitalization is necessary).

2. During the period of mood disturbance, three (or more) of the following symptoms have persisted (four if the mood is only irritable) and have been present to a significant degree:
   - Inflated self-esteem or grandiosity
   - Decreased need for sleep (e.g. feels rested after only three hours of sleep)
   - More talkative than usual or pressure to keep talking
   - Flight of ideas or subjective experience that thoughts are racing
   - Distractibility (i.e. attention too easily drawn to unimportant or irrelevant external stimuli)
   - Increase in goal-directed activity (either socially, at work or school, or sexually) or psychomotor agitation
   - Excessive involvement in pleasurable activities that have a high potential for painful consequences (e.g. engaging in unrestrained buying sprees, sexual indiscretions, or foolish business investments)

3. The symptoms do not meet criteria for a mixed episode

4. The mood disturbance is sufficiently severe to cause marked impairment in occupational functioning or in usual social activities or relationships with others, or to necessitate hospitalization to prevent harm to self or to others, or there are psychotic features

5. The symptoms are not due to the direct physiological effects of a substance (e.g. drug of abuse, a medication, or other treatment) or a general medical condition (e.g. hypothyroidism).

often impaired during a manic episode and can result in indiscreet or dangerous behaviour ranging from overspending and being sexually inappropriate to unnecessary risk taking and self harm. Further, because of mania, individuals often indulge in excessive substance misuse, especially alcohol and occasionally become intrusive or aggressive and sometimes can not control their behaviour. In addition to these experiences, it is not unusual for patients with mania to have inflated self esteem and feel they are special or have grandiose and delusional ideas. Indeed, when mania is severe, it often melds into psychosis.

2.1.1.2 *Hypomania*

This term is used to describe a 'milder' form of mania where only some of the symptoms of mania occur. Further, the individual does not have hallucinations or delusions (is not psychotic). The symptoms may alter functioning but overall functioning is not significantly impaired and hence hospitalization is not usually required for the treatment of hypomania. In practice hypomania can be difficult to diagnose because the symptoms can be subtle or fail to register as problematic. Not surprisingly, patients rarely present complaining of hypomanic symptoms. However, hypomania can be a precursor to mania and is important to detect as it can alter the diagnosis from major depression to that of Bipolar II disorder.

2.1.1.3 *Bipolar depressive episode*

In bipolar depression individuals experience a qualitative change in mood that results in feelings of sadness, hopelessness and self blame that are sometimes accompanied by anxiety and anger. These symptoms usually occur alongside changes in levels of energy most commonly, fatigue and listlessness, with a lack of interest in activities that the individual would normally enjoy (anhedonia). Changes in sleep and appetite with difficulties in concentrating are coupled with a lack of motivation and a loss of interest in intimacy. In addition, individuals often develop suicidal thoughts and in severe cases may experience psychotic symptoms such as delusions and hallucinations. The risk of suicide is high in bipolar depressed patients. Typically, the features of bipolar depression are more melancholic than those of unipolar major depression with a greater likelihood of psychomotor retardation and atypical symptoms such as hypersomnia.

The criteria for a major depressive episode in bipolar disorder are essentially the same as those of major (unipolar) depression. (see Box 2.2). A diagnosis of bipolar depression requires that five or more of the key symptoms are present for more than two weeks but this means that in any particular individual the profile of bipolar depressive symptoms can vary considerably.

2.1.1.4 *Mixed affective episodes (mixed states)*

Mixed states are even more difficult to diagnose than hypomania but are important as they are common in clinical practice, and cause significant disability. Mixed episodes are in essence periods of mood disturbance that last at least one week during which the symptoms of *both* clinical depression and mania occur simultaneously. These patients typically have dysphoria, irritability and increased anxiety, agitation along with other symptoms of depression and mania. Subsets of mixed states have been identified and described, such as dysphoric mania, mixed mania or mixed depression so as to reflect the predominance of one pole or another. However, clinically these subdivisions are of limited use as they do not meaningfully inform treatment.

Box 2.2 DSM-IV criteria for depression

Five (or more) of the following symptoms have been present during the same two-week period and represent a change from previous functioning: at least one of the symptoms is either (1) depressed mood or (2) loss of interest of pleasure. Note: do not include symptoms that are clearly due to a general medical conditional or mood-incongruent delusions or hallucinations.

• Depressed mood most of the day, nearly every day, as indicated by either subjective report (e.g. feels sad or empty) or observation made by others (e.g. appears tearful). Note: in children and adolescents, can be irritable mood

• Markedly diminished interest or pleasure in all, or almost all, activities most of the day, nearly every day (as indicated by either subjective account or observation made by others)

• Significant weight loss when not dieting or weight gain (e.g. change of more than 5% of body weight in a month), or decrease or increase in appetite nearly every day. In children, consider failure to make expected weight gains

• Insomnia or hypersomnia nearly every day

• Psychomotor agitation or retardation nearly every day (observable by others not merely subjective feelings or restlessness or being slowed down)

• Fatigue or loss of energy nearly every day

• Feelings of worthlessness or excessive or inappropriate guilt (which may be delusional) nearly every day (not merely self-reproach or guilt about being sick)

• Diminished ability to think or concentrate, or indecisiveness, nearly every day (either by subjective account or as observed by others)

• Recurrent thoughts of death (not just fear of dying), recurrent suicidal ideation without a specific plan, or a suicide attempt or a specific plan for committing suicide.

Note: The symptoms do not meet criteria for a mixed episode; cause clinically significant distress or impairment in social, occupational, or other important areas of functioning; are not due to the direct physiological effects of a substance or general medical condition and are not better accounted for by bereavement.

2.1.2 Diagnoses

The two main classification systems that are used to define neuropsychiatric disorders for research and clinical practice are ICD-10 and DSM-IV. The latter is more widely adopted and so for simplicity we refer here only to DSM-IV. The classification of bipolar disorder according to DSM-IV is shown in Figure 2.1. Subtypes can be identified

Figure 2.1 Bipolar disorder diagnoses

BIPOLAR I Presence of at least one episode of mania with a minimum duration of one week with or without major depressive episodes.	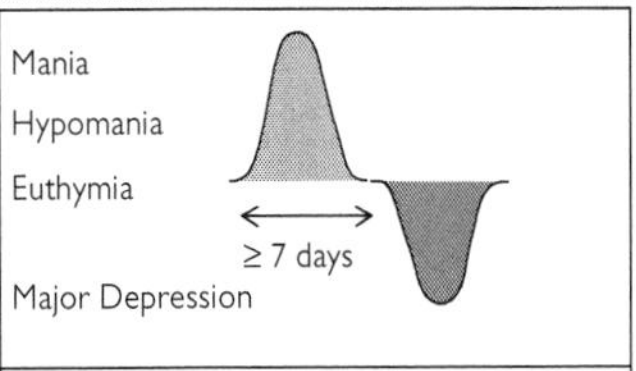 Mania Hypomania Euthymia ≥ 7 days Major Depression
BIPOLAR II Presence of one or more episodes of hypomania accompanied by at least one episode of major depression with no psychotic features.	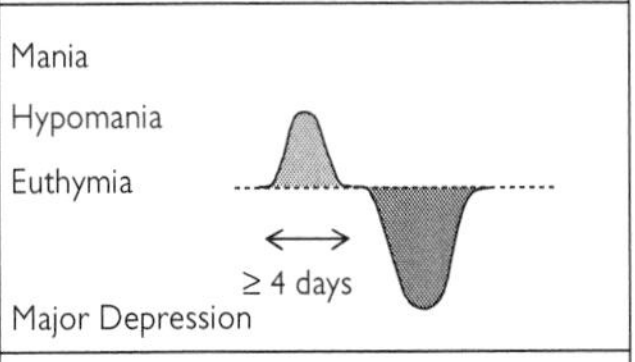 Mania Hypomania Euthymia ≥ 4 days Major Depression
CYCLOTHYMIA One or more episodes of hypomania and periods of depressive symptoms that do not meet criteria for a major depressive episode.	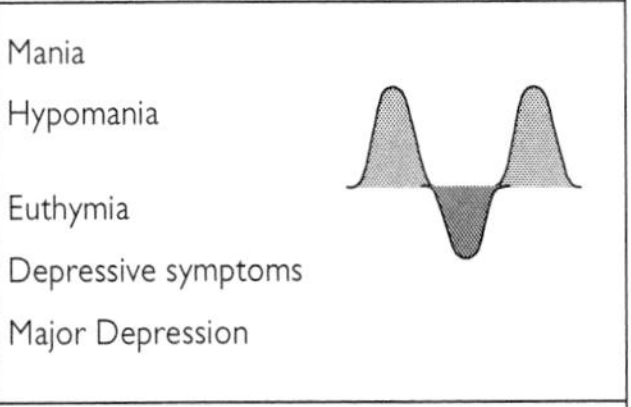 Mania Hypomania Euthymia Depressive symptoms Major Depression
RAPID CYCLING The occurrence of four or more episodes of depression or mania during 12 months. Episodes can occur in any combination or order but must satisfy duration & symptom criteria for Major Depression, Mania or Hypomania and must be separated by either a period of remission or by a switch to the opposite pole (for at least 2 months) of illness.	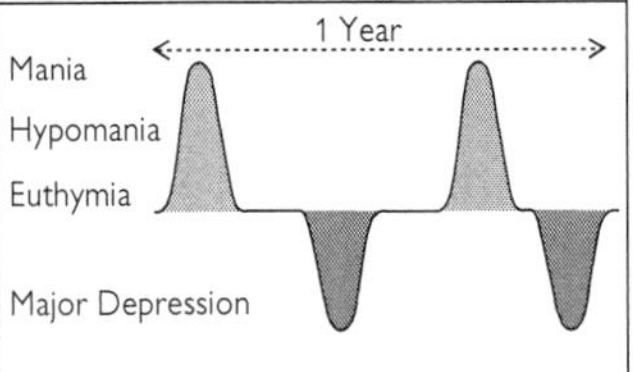 1 Year Mania Hypomania Euthymia Major Depression
MIXED EPISODES Concurrent symptoms of depression and mania. Mania plus at least two of six dysphoric symptoms: anhedonia, guilt, depressed mood, anxiety, fatigue, suicidal ideation.	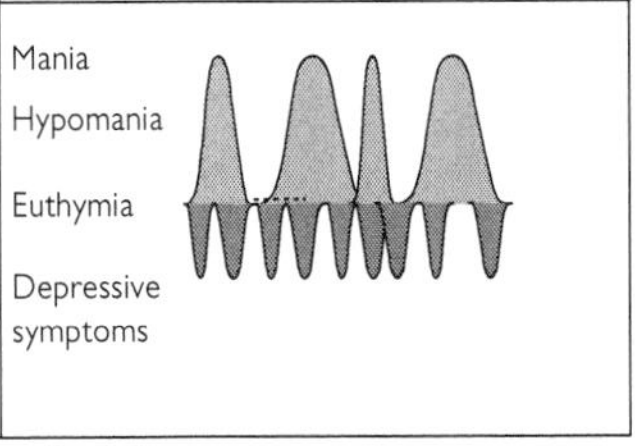 Mania Hypomania Euthymia Depressive symptoms

* Adapted from DSM-IV-TR and Malhi & Berk (2008), and simplified for clarity.

by using a clinical interview and examination that relies on DSM-IV criteria or a more sophisticated assessment such as a structured clinical interview for DSM diagnosis (SCID) can be used to appraise complex clinical presentations. A careful assessment is usually necessary to confidently diagnose bipolar disorder subtypes.

In practice, patients with bipolar disorder seek help mainly during depressive episodes which are often clinically indistinguishable from major depression. The diagnosis of bipolar disorder is therefore often delayed. Further, current classifications do not completely reflect the myriad of presentations found in clinical practice that include, for instance, subsyndromal symptoms and treatment-induced mood changes. These additional 'forms' of bipolar disorder are broadly grouped as bipolar disorder not otherwise specified (Bipolar NOS). In addition to Bipolar NOS, DSM-IV describes Bipolar I disorder, Bipolar II disorder and cyclothymia.

2.1.2.1 *Bipolar I*

For a diagnosis of bipolar I disorder an individual has to have experienced one or more manic or mixed episodes. This can occur with or without a major depressive episode though in most cases depression is a significant component of the illness.

2.1.2.2 *Bipolar II*

In bipolar II disorder the individual has never experienced a manic or mixed episode. Instead the individual has hypomanic episodes in addition to at least one major depressive episode. Typically, hypomanic episodes are less severe than mania with less severe occupational and social impairment. Further, in hypomania there is no psychosis and there is usually no need to hospitalize the individual. However, the diagnostic criteria are somewhat arbitrary and the symptoms can often be difficult to distinguish from normal changes in behavior, mood and thinking. The diagnosis of bipolar II disorder is therefore more difficult to make reliably than bipolar I disorder.

2.1.2.3 *Cyclothymia*

In cyclothymic disorder the individual experiences numerous hypomanic episodes that are interspersed with periods of depressive symptoms that do not meet the full criteria for a major depressive episode. In essence, cyclothymia describes low grade cycling of mood that may result in changes in function.

2.1.2.4 *Bipolar not otherwise specified (bipolar NOS)*

As described above this is not a diagnostic category *per se* but a term that is intended to capture presentations that do not fit neatly into other diagnostic categories.

2.1.2.5 *Course specifiers*

A number of terms are used to describe the course of bipolar illness such as catatonia, melancholia, chronic and rapid cycling. Of these rapid cycling is most widely used and can be applied to any of the subtypes of bipolar disorder. Rapid cycling is defined as having *four or more episodes of mood disturbance per year* (major depression, mania, hypomania or mixed episode). Of note, terms used to describe even more frequent shifts in mood have been introduced into the literature such as ultra-rapid and ultra-ultra or ultradian cycling that reflect the more frequent and shorter mood episode cycles in bipolar disorder.

2.2 Screening and diagnostic assessment

Ideally a definitive diagnosis of bipolar disorder should be made by a mental health professional such as a psychiatrist. However, other than extreme manifestations of mania that present to the hospital, the illness usually emerges gradually and is first observed in a community setting. Therefore most early encounters involve primary care physicians and hence a number of useful screening instruments have been developed that can be completed through self-report or administered by the clinician (see Chapter 9). It is important to note however that these instruments serve only as a screen and are not designed to be diagnostic. A definitive diagnosis of bipolar disorder usually requires a comprehensive clinical assessment and medical evaluation. This is particularly important when assessing bipolar symptoms as many of these can be caused by an organic illness and therefore ideally all patients suspected of a mood disorder should be screened at the outset for organic causes of mood disturbance.

2.3 Differential diagnosis and comorbidity of bipolar disorder

2.3.1 Major depression

The differential diagnosis of bipolar disorder is relatively broad, partly because the manifestations of the illness are quite varied. Depressive episodes are more common than manic/hypomanic episodes in bipolar disorder and are more distressing to the patients. Hence, patients with bipolar disorder seek help mainly during depressive episodes. Given that the symptoms of bipolar depression and unipolar depression are similar, these patients are routinely misdiagnosed as unipolar (major) depression.

We recommend that all patients presenting with depressive symptoms should be routinely screened for a previous history of symptoms of mania. Questions related to periods of decreased sleep, racing thoughts and increased energy are more sensitive in eliciting previous manic episodes than screening for a period of euphoric mood. Further, features of depression that are more common and favor a diagnosis of bipolar depression are listed in Table 2.2. Clinically, these are of some value but a high index of suspicion is often needed and in addition it is important to monitor the response to antidepressant treatment. Generally, bipolar depression is less responsive to antidepressants than unipolar depression and is more likely to switch into treatment-induced mania, a mixed state or develop a rapid cycling pattern of mood.

2.3.1.1 *Anxiety disorders*
Virtually all patients with bipolar disorder experience significant anxiety symptoms at some stage during the course of their illness. Estimates and population data suggest that 75–90% of patients with bipolar I disorder have comorbid clinical anxiety and in practice anxiety symptoms are often the first to manifest. The anxiety disorders that are commonly found in patients with bipolar disorder are panic and generalized anxiety disorder. However, obsessive compulsive disorder is also reported in significant numbers and in many cases of bipolar disorder it is the symptoms of anxiety that the individual finds most troubling.

2.3.1.2 *Substance misuse*

Patients with both bipolar I, and bipolar II disorder have clinically significant comorbid substance misuse. Most frequent is the abuse of alcohol but illicit substance use is also common and this usually includes drugs such as cannabis, cocaine, ecstasy and amphetamines. The excessive use of addictive drugs perhaps occurs partly because of their ability to transiently lift mood and alleviate anxiety.

Table 2.2 Features of depression that suggest a diagnosis of bipolar depression rather than unipolar (major) depression	
Signs and symptoms:	Irritability
	Melancholia
	Psychotic symptoms during depression
	Psychomotor changes
	Atypical symptoms such as hypersomnia and hyperphagia
Pattern of illness:	Early age of onset
	Recurrent brief episodes
	Multiple episodes
	Family history of bipolar disorder

Patients with primary substance abuse may also present with mood symptoms that mimic bipolar disorder. Family history of bipolar disorder and presence of mood symptoms in the absence of substance use may favour the diagnosis of bipolar disorder. Further, those with primary substance abuse tend to abuse multiple drugs while those with bipolar disorder tend to stick to one or two drugs such as alcohol or cocaine.

It is important to recognize and appropriately manage comorbid substance misuse disorders because they are greatly disruptive in their own right but also contribute indirectly to the chaos of bipolar disorder. Suitable treatment of comorbid substance misuse enhances bipolar disorder treatment compliance and improves overall clinical outcome. Often this necessitates the involvement of specialized services and depending upon the severity of the substance misuse, this may need to be prioritized.

2.3.2 Borderline personality disorder

Borderline personality disorder shares many features with bipolar disorder for instance marked mood instability and impulsivity. Therefore it is not surprising that clinically the two diagnoses often overlap. To complicate the matters further, borderline personality disorder is comorbid with bipolar disorder in about 20 to 30% of bipolar patients. From a diagnostic perspective (in particular DSM-IV) both diagnoses (Axis I and Axis II) can be applied concurrently. Patients with borderline personality disorder tend to have a history of abuse, chaotic relationships, mood instability and no period of prolonged normal functioning. True euphoria is rare in borderline personality disorder. A family history of bipolar disorder, some clear euthymic intervals, euphoria and manic episodes support the diagnosis of bipolar disorder.

2.3.3 Schizophrenia

Patients presenting with first episode mania often have psychotic symptoms, excitability and agitation and therefore, they are often misdiagnosed as having a brief psychotic episode or schizophreniform psychosis. Family history of schizophrenia, premorbid personality difficulties, bizarre psychotic symptoms, poorer functioning prior to the onset of psychotic symptoms as well as lack of any significant and pervasive mood symptoms suggests a diagnosis of schizophrenia. When unclear, prospective observation and mood monitoring might help.

In recent years the term psychosis has been used to describe symptoms without referring to a diagnosis per se. The 'category' therefore subsumes presentations that are as yet diagnostically equivocal but allows treatment to be commenced with a focus on symptomatic improvement and clinical care. Once a definitive diagnosis emerges management can be adapted accordingly.

2.3.4 Organic causes

General medical conditions often produce symptoms that appear to mimic depression, mania, or psychosis. The range of disorders that can cause psychological changes akin to bipolar disorder is extensive and includes neurological conditions, infectious diseases, endocrine disorders (in particular thyroid disease) and iatrogenic causes such as the administration of medications. An organic cause for bipolar disorder should be considered in every new presentation of bipolar disorder. Therefore the assessment of patients with bipolar disorder must include a comprehensive physical examination, drug screen, hematological and biochemical evaluation. In instances where a neurological cause is suspected, a brain scan such as a CT or MRI may be warranted.

2.4 Assigning a diagnosis of bipolar disorder

In practice, the key distinction to be made is that between bipolar disorder and major depression because this has clear treatment implications. Clinically, this means that it is important to maintain a reasonably high degree of suspicion for bipolar disorder but at the same time have a high threshold for ultimately assigning the diagnosis. This is because the impact of the diagnosis on the individual and their family is likely to be significant as it has many consequences for future employment, relationships and personal aspirations and goals. It is also important to ensure that the individual understands the implications of the diagnosis and has a clear appreciation of what to expect. In particular the fact that bipolar disorder is a chronic illness that will require careful life long management is an important message to communicate soon after diagnosis. Assignment of the diagnosis should therefore, where possible, involve key family members and significant others who also need to be aware of the nature of the illness and understand their potential role in management

References and further reading

American Psychiatric Association (2000). *Diagnostic and statistical manual for mental disorders*, 4th edn, text revision (DSM-IV-TR). Washington, DC: American Psychiatric Association.

Angst J, Sellaro R (2000). Historical perspectives and natural history of bipolar disorder. *Biological Psychiatry*, **48**(6), 445–57.

Goodwin FK, Jamison K (2007). *Manic-depressive illness: Bipolar disorders and recurrent depression*. 2nd ed. New York: Oxford University Press.

Malhi GS, Berk M (2009). How to treat bipolar disorder. *Australian Doctor* 2008 [cited 14th April]; available from: www.australiandoctor.com.au.

World Health Organisation (1992). *The ICD-10 classification of mental and behavioural disorders: clinical description and diagnostic guidelines.* Geneva: WHO.

Yatham LN (2005). Diagnosis and management of patients with bipolar II disorder. *Journal of Clinical Psychiatry*, **66**(1), 13–17.

Chapter 3

Epidemiology

Key points

- Bipolar I and Bipolar II disorder each affect approximately 1% of the population
- Bipolar disorder affects males and females equally
- Bipolar disorder emerges early in life, typically below the age of 20 years
- Bipolar disorder is a chronic episodic illness and up to 15% of patients commit suicide.

3.1 Epidemiology

The lifetime prevalence rates of bipolar disorder vary depending upon the methods used. A recent estimate suggests that bipolar I disorder affects approximately 1% and bipolar II disorder 1.1% of the population. Sub-threshold cases that meet some, but not all, of the necessary criteria for these subtypes, are thought to contribute an additional 2 to 5% and therefore collectively as much as 4 to 7% of individuals may qualify as having a disorder that falls within the 'bipolar spectrum'.

In recent years there has been speculation that the prevalence of bipolar disorder has increased, however whether this is true remains unclear. The increase in diagnosis of bipolar disorder worldwide may be attributable to a number of factors other than an increase in the incidence of the illness *per se* such as, an increasing awareness of bipolar disorder amongst the general population and better detection by health care professionals.

It is of note that the detection and diagnosis of bipolar disorder at a young age is largely a USA phenomenon. North American child and adolescent psychiatrists are virtually alone in assigning a diagnosis of bipolar disorder to children less than 10 years of age. This is seldom observed elsewhere in the world. This increase in paediatric bipolar disorder that is peculiar to the USA may reflect the use of broader diagnostic criteria or may be a consequence of the widespread use of stimulants that are administered to children to manage hyperactivity.

3.2 Demographic and social factors

3.2.1 Gender

In contrast to unipolar (major) depression, which is clearly more prevalent in women than in men with a gender ratio of at least two to one, bipolar disorder is equally common across the sexes though this is probably only accurate for bipolar I disorder. For other sub-types, such as bipolar II disorder and rapid cycling bipolar disorder, there appears to be a gender bias towards females. Hence, across the spectrum of mood disorders (bipolar I and bipolar II disorder to unipolar depression) the increasing prevalence amongst women is linked to the rate of depression.

3.2.2 Age and ethnicity

The age of onset of bipolar disorder is significantly younger than un-ipolar (major) depression with the illness emerging most commonly between the ages of 12 and 20 years. Bipolar II disorder appears to have a slightly later age of onset than bipolar I disorder and generally a younger age of onset in bipolar disorder has been associated with a family history of bipolarity. In the majority of patients, bipolar disorder initially presents with an episode of depression and though an initial onset with a manic episode is not uncommon, it becomes less likely with increasing age.

A diagnosis of bipolar disorder is often made during late adolescence and early adulthood with a clear onset of symptoms during the teenage years. This is a critical time for physiological growth and behavioral change. During this time the brain undergoes extensive cognitive development and the individual experiences a marked social and emotional transformation. Against this evolving background the signs and symptoms of bipolar disorder are easily overlooked. These physiological changes can therefore mask the disorder but can at the same time be disrupted by the illness or by treatments that are administered to manage the symptoms.

Interestingly, the prevalence of bipolar disorder does not seem to be dependent upon ethnicity. It is likely that perceived differences across different societies reflect cultural differences that affect awareness and the identification of the illness. Economic and political differences are important factors that likely influence the provision of services and the choice of diagnoses made available to doctors. For instance, in many countries medications that are not indicated for bipolar disorder cannot be prescribed under government reimbursement schemes unless a firm diagnosis of bipolar disorder has been established. Even with a confirmed diagnosis there are often restrictions because of economic reasons as to which medications can be prescribed. In contrast in some societies suitable medications may be available but the individual and their family are often not accepting of the diagnosis and will only engage services or take medication if it is prescribed for general health reasons such as treating 'stress'.

3.2.3 Marital status and socioeconomic factors

Marital and socioeconomic status is invariably found to be associated with bipolar disorder. However, because these factors are complex and multidimensional it is difficult to determine causality. For instance, divorce or separation can both contribute to and be the effect of the illness, and similarly unemployment can lead to the precipitation of bipolar disorder or arise as a consequence of the illness.

3.3 Course of bipolar disorder

3.3.1 Pattern of Illness

Initially, manic-depressive illness was thought to have a relatively good prognosis and this is probably true for 'classic bipolar disorder'. However, the majority of bipolar patients with episodes of mania and depression, or an admixture of mood disturbance, do not have a classic form of the illness and many do not achieve full functional recovery. Indeed in recent years it has become increasingly evident that the course of bipolar disorder is more chronic and extremely variable. Many patients have mixed episodes, or periods of extended mood disturbance in which individual episodes are difficult to identify. Some individuals with bipolar disorder swing and switch from one pole of the illness to the other several times in one year resulting in rapid cycling presentations, whereas others experience even more frequent switching that can result in several significant mood changes within a single day. These unstable forms of the illness are necessarily harder to treat and extremely distressing to the individuals affected. Further, sub-syndromal symptoms are very common in bipolar patients in treatment.

3.3.2 Outcome of bipolar disorder

Bipolar disorder is a recurrent episodic illness that is characterized by periods of spontaneous remission that can lead to recovery or relapse. Untreated, episodes of mania typically last an average of six to 12 weeks and episodes of bipolar depression last approximately 12 to 24 weeks. About two thirds of patients with bipolar disorder usually recover within six months following an episode of depression or mania but up to 5% may not recover within five years. Non-response is more likely with mixed episodes or a cycling pattern of illness.

Chronic subsyndromal symptoms cause considerable functional impairment and are common with up to a third of patients reporting extended periods of being persistently unwell. Predictors of poor outcome include personality disorders, comorbid substance misuse, and predominance of depressive symptoms, poor inter-episode recovery and poor treatment compliance. A rapid cycling pattern of illness is also a poor prognostic factor as is the occurrence of mixed affective episodes and psychotic symptoms.

Recent findings suggest that episodes of bipolar illness may have a cumulative effect on the brain and that long-term patients with bipolar disorder may experience significant cognitive compromise.

3.3.3 Suicide

Suicide is a significant risk factor for patients with bipolar disorder occurring in particular during depressive episodes and mixed states. In the most severely affected bipolar patients, namely those admitted to hospital, the suicide rate is approximately 15% and thus contributes disproportionately to the increased mortality associated with the illness. Treatment and compliance with treatment along with the establishment of a therapeutic relationship are important protective factors. Amongst the medications lithium in particular has been shown to have unique anti-suicidal properties.

References and further reading

Bauer M, Pfennig A (2005). Epidemiology of bipolar disorders. *Epilepsia*, **46**(4): 8–13.

Kessler RC, Berglund P, Demler O, Jin R, Merikangas KR, Walters EE (2005). Lifetime prevalence and age-of-onset distributions of DSM-IV disorders in the National Comorbidity Survey Replication. *Archives of General Psychiatry*, **62**(6), 593–602.

Merikangas KR, Akiskal HS, Angst J, Greenberg PE, Hirschfeld RM, Petukhova M et al. (2007). Lifetime and 12-month prevalence of bipolar spectrum disorder in the National Comorbidity Survey Replication, *Archives of General Psychiatry*, **64**(5), 543–52.

Tohen M, Bromet E, Murphy JM, Tsuang MT (2000). Psychiatric epidemiology, *Harvard Review of Psychiatry*, **8**(3), 111–25.

Chapter 4

The causes of bipolar disorder

Key points

- Bipolar disorder is the most heritable psychiatric disorder
- Environmental factors can contribute to the onset and development of mood episodes
- Structural and functional brain changes along with neuroendocrine and neurocognitive changes have been identified in bipolar disorder
- Bipolar disorder has a neurobiological basis but its detailed pathophysiology is unknown.

4.1 Introduction

Bipolar disorder usually emerges in adolescence and early adulthood, a stage in life marked by change. As discussed in Chapter 2, this can make early and accurate diagnosis challenging. In broad terms, bipolar disorder is more heritable than unipolar (major) depression. It is important to note, that although there is likely a significant genetic predisposition in most cases, strong environmental factors play a role in the onset and development of the illness. However, the exact mechanisms by which these factors ultimately contribute to the manifestation of signs and symptoms, remains unclear.

This chapter provides a brief overview of factors currently thought to contribute to the development of bipolar disorder.

4.2 Genetic causes

Bipolar disorder is one of the most heritable psychiatric disorders, and often runs in families. Broadly speaking, the risk of bipolar I disorder in the families (first degree relatives) of patients with the illness is nearly ten-fold the risk in the general population. It is therefore no surprise that if one twin is affected by bipolar disorder the other has a substantial likelihood of developing the illness. Specifically, the concordance rate for monozygotic twins (twins that have the same genes) is approximately 40–70% whereas the rate for dizygotic twins is much less and ranges from 10%–20%. It is worth highlighting that the concordance rate in monozygotic twins is *not* 100%, indicating that other factors play a significant role. Figures for bipolar II disorder are lower, and the heritability of bipolar disorder probably overlaps to some extent with that of unipolar depression and psychosis. Overall, bipolar disorder is a complex disorder and its heritability is likely to be determined by a number of related genes, rather than a single gene defect. This raises the intriguing possibility that there are different sub-types of bipolar disorder with a differing genetic makeup.

Over the past two decades genetic studies have identified many chromosomal regions and potential genes (*candidate genes*) that appear to be associated with the development of bipolar disorder. Although many genes have been implicated and various genes have been associated with bipolar disorder in different families, no single gene or single locus has been unequivocally linked to bipolar disorder. In fact, many findings await replication and strong associations are yet to be consistently identified.

These diverse findings strongly point to heterogeneity within the illness. It is now widely accepted that bipolar disorder is most likely a polygenic disease that is complex in its pattern of heritability. There is thought to be an interaction between genes that confer risk and those that are possibly protective, with environmental factors also impacting the expression of genetic information. The methodologies that have been used to study the genetics of bipolar disorder are complicated; they are summarized in brief in Table 4.1.

A synthesis of the findings from numerous linkage and association studies suggests that genes related to neurotransmitter function such as dopamine (DRD IV and SLC 683), serotonin (SLC 6A4 and TPH 2), and glutamate (DAOA and DTNBP1), and others related to cellular physiology (BDNF, DISC1 and NRG1), are of salience in the pathophysiology of bipolar disorder. Other regions of interest involving chromosomes (16p12 locus) and genes (GHKH and ANK3) have been identified through genome wide association analyses and these genes have been found to have a role in the transmission of intracellular information and the regulation of ion channels. Of particular interest is the potential role of mitochondria that regulate intracellular calcium and synaptic plasticity. A range of methodologies including genetic studies have implicated mitochondrial dysfunction in bipolar disorder. These studies have found that changes in neuronal metabolism and intracellular calcium levels affect gene transcription, and that genes such as brain derived neurotophic factor (BDNF) are dependent on neuronal activity and are implicated in mood disorders. However, despite all these insights the current consensus is that individual genes

Table 4.1 Research methodologies used in bipolar disorder genetic research				
	Linkage studies	Association studies	Genome wide association studies	Pathways based analysis
Data	Bipolar individuals and their family members (siblings, parents)	Groups of patients with bipolar disorder and healthy controls	Groups of patients with bipolar disorder and healthy controls	Linkage, association and genome wide association studies data is pooled and correlated with other information
Method	Examine the pattern of inheritance of specific chromosomal fragments across relatives so as to identify common regions associated with the disorder	Compare gene variants in large samples of affected and unaffected individuals	Involves a whole genome scan across all chromosomes of bipolar disorder patients in a group to identify common gene variants	More sophisticated analyses that examine more than simple associations and correlations

are likely to have a relatively small effect and that although the overall genetic contribution to BD is significant it ultimately constitutes a complex set of genetic vulnerabilities.

4.3 Environmental causes

Clinically, it is clear that environmental factors influence the development of bipolar disorder. Research suggests that psychosocial events may contribute both directly and via interactions with genetic factors. Recently, it has been shown that life events—and in particular factors pertaining to interpersonal relationships—can influence both onset and relapse. Further, tracing etiological factors back to childhood reveals that a significant proportion of adults with bipolar disorder identify experiences of trauma and abuse that perhaps relate to earlier onset and greater comorbidity. The exact mechanisms by which environmental factors result in the development of mood episodes or cause bipolar illness remain unclear. Life events such as losses and periods of stress have been shown to be significant factors in the development and manifestation of unipolar depression; however, their role in bipolar disorder is less clear.

Kraepelin was perhaps the first to suggest that initial episodes of bipolar depression or mania were closely associated with psychosocial stressors. This idea of 'stress sensitization' has been borne out to some extent in subsequent research, but data also indicate that the necessity for stress to precipitate episodes diminishes as the illness progresses, and that ultimately episodes of bipolar disorder can occur spontaneously.

4.4 Neurobiological causes

Although an extensive body of research has examined the biological abnormalities associated with bipolar depression and mania, a comprehensive model has not emerged. Many findings relate to the acute phases of the illness but are not unique to bipolar disorder and as such may be epiphenomena. Recent bipolar disorder research has increasingly focused on the euthymic phase of the illness along with its onset and relapsing nature, and this seems to be a more promising approach for identifying potentially core deficits. A number of neurobiological domains have been investigated; those that have provided some promising insights are briefly considered here.

4.4.1 Neurochemistry of bipolar disorder

Early research focused predominantly on the neurochemistry of bipolar disorder largely because of the monoamine hypothesis of depression and the serendipitous discovery of effective psychotropic medications.

4.4.1.1 *Bipolar depression*

The neurotransmitter that has been most widely implicated in the pathophysiology of depression is serotonin. Unipolar depression research examining serotonergic neurotransmitter pathways and the metabolism of serotonin suggests that it has a pivotal role in depression. Further, medications such as the selective serotonin reuptake inhibitors (SSRIs) and others that enhance serotonergic function have proved to be successful antidepressants in the short term treatment of major (unipolar) depression. In addition, individuals that recover from depression can be neurochemically manipulated to develop depressive symptoms by limiting the availability of tryptophan, a substrate for serotonin. However, in bipolar I disorder similar research involving tryptophan depletion has failed to show a strong link between serotonin and bipolar depression. This weaker association is perhaps reflected by the lack of consistent efficacy of antidepressants in the treatment of bipolar depression as compared to major depression. Therefore, in addition to the monoamines, other neurotransmitters are likely to be of importance in the pathophysiology of bipolar depression such as GABA and glutamate. Research examining these neurotransmitters is still in its early phases but has been assisted greatly by brain imaging techniques such as proton spectroscopy that assess the concentration of these molecules in vivo.

4.4.1.2 *Mania*

In contrast to depression, mania appears to be more strongly underpinned by dopaminergic dysfunction. Amphetamine, a psychotomimetic, can induce euphoria and other cognitive and behavioural changes in healthy individuals that are similar to mania, and precipitate manic episodes in those with a history or vulnerability to bipolar disorder. Its primary action is the release of dopamine and other monoamines, and it generally increases neurotransmitter turnover, in particular that of dopamine.

The dopamine pathways implicated in bipolar disorder connect the frontal cortex and striatum, and the depletion of dopamine precursors such as tyrosine and phenylalanine is antimanic. Dopaminergic over-activity in mania is further indicated by the antimanic efficacy of atypical antipsychotics, which have been shown to produce dopamine D2 receptor blockade. Recent positron emission tomography (PET) studies suggest that mood stabilizers such as valproate, which are antimanic, reduce dopamine turnover, and that manic patients may release increased dopamine into synaptic space compared with healthy controls, thus supporting the dopamine hyperactivity theory of mania. However, like bipolar depression a single neurotransmitter does not provide a complete explanation for the pathophysiology of mania. There is growing interest in the role of additional neurotransmitters such as glutamate and other excitatory amino acids.

4.4.2 Molecular and cellular findings

Lithium and valproate are commonly used mood stabilizers in the treatment of bipolar disorder (see Chapter 7). They are thought to act via modulation of intracellular targets as opposed to actions on cell surface receptors. A number of putative intracellular targets have been identified and the findings in relation to these targets are briefly summarized.

At clinically therapeutic concentrations lithium competes with magnesium and inhibits a number of key enzymes. These enzymes are involved in a number of cellular signalling systems such as the phosphoinositol and Wnt pathways.

The phosphoinositol (PI) cascade is a G-protein regulated signalling pathway that has been widely studied in bipolar disorder. Lithium directly inhibits the enzymes inositol monophosphatase (IMPase) and inositol polyphosphate 1-phosphatase (IPPase) and thereby diminishes the availability of myoinositol. This results in inositol depletion and subsequently the depletion of PI and is thought to ultimately disrupt the second messenger signalling pathway. Although this is an attractive and plausible mechanism for the actions of lithium, preliminary findings do not fully support this model, and the focus of research has shifted to downstream targets such as protein kinase C (PKC) isoenzymes. Interestingly, valproate also inhibits PKC signaling and agents that precipitate mania have the opposite effect. Therefore centrally acting PKC inhibitors such as tamoxifen may exert antimanic effects via this cellular mechanism.

GSK3 is implicated in the regulation of synaptic plasticity and has been shown to antagonize both insulin and Wnt signalling pathways. The inhibition of GSK3 by lithium may therefore explain its ability to enhance neuronal growth, modify synaptogenesis and stimulate neurogensis in the hippocampus. However, at therapeutic doses of lithium the model only holds partly, and the mechanisms of intracellular signalling and the effects of secondary GSK3 inhibition remain to be fully elucidated.

In addition to its acute effects on intracellular molecules, chronic lithium administration induces neuroprotective and neurotrophic proteins. These include BDNF and Bcl-2. The latter is a neuroprotective protein that can also stimulate neuronal regeneration, whereas BDNF is strongly implicated in adult hippocampal neurogenesis and the regulation of mood and antidepressant treatment responsivity. These roles and potential cellular effects of lithium are reflected clinically. Recent studies have shown that lithium is neuroprotective across a number of neuropsychiatric illnesses including bipolar disorder, and that chronic lithium administration in bipolar disorder increases regional gray matter volume and can produce an increase in the N-acetyl aspartate (NAA) that serves as a marker of neuronal viability.

In sum the findings from molecular studies are providing exciting insights into the cellular pathophysiology of bipolar disorder and the putative mechanisms of action of mood stabilizing medications such as lithium and valproate. Better understanding is likely to yield additional treatment targets for novel mood-stabilizing agents. However, the cellular models for bipolar disorder do not fully explain the etiology of the illness and the therapeutic effects of medications and therefore require considerable further investigation and testing.

4.4.3 Neuroendocrine findings

Neuroendocrine changes have been noted in mood disorders for many years. The most intriguing observation has been that of raised plasma cortisol found in patients with bipolar disorder during both mania and severe depression. Interestingly, with clinical recovery cortisol levels eventually normalize suggesting that neuroendocrine change is somehow related to the onset or manifestation of the disorder. This finding has been investigated by manipulating normally occurring feedback within the hypothalamic-adrenal (HPA) axis using dexamethasone (a glucocorticoid). The administration of dexamethasone usually leads to the suppression of cortisol release, and a failure to suppress (non-suppression) cortisol release is deemed abnormal. Hypercortisolaemia has been found in severe major (unipolar) depression and in euthymic bipolar disorder. In major depression this and other HPA axis abnormalities have been linked to adrenal gland enlargement. However, the implications for bipolar disorder are less clear. In healthy subjects and in patients with bipolar I disorder the exogenous administration of cortisol can readily produce mood changes and induce mania. Interestingly, long-term use of cortisol usually leads to a depressive syndrome and therefore many investigators are researching the possibility that cortisol antagonism may yield antidepressant or even antimanic effects.

The other major hormone that contributes to mood and is sometimes found to be altered in bipolar disorder is thyroxine. This hormone is produced and released by the thyroid gland. Thyroxine deficiency (hypothyroidism) produces mood symptoms similar to clinical depression, whereas an excess of this hormone can lead to hyperthyroidism that is usually characterized by emotional instability, anxiety and agitation. Of note, rapid cycling bipolar I disorder and bipolar depression have been associated with mild hypothyroidism and in some cases the administration of thyroid hormones has been shown to be of some benefit. However, the picture in bipolar disorder is confounded somewhat by the fact that lithium disrupts thyroid function and lowers circulating thyroid hormone levels. Therefore, about 10% of patients with long term lithium therapy develop hypothyroidism.

Although neuroendocrine changes noted in bipolar disorder are incompletely understood, they provide a potential link between environmental psychosocial stressors and events and the neurobiology of the illness. In particular, the HPA axis is implicated in mediating stress related signals to and from the brain and may be the conduit by which stressful life events result in hormonal and subsequent neurobiological changes that eventually lead to mood dysfunction.

4.4.4 Neuroimaging and neuropsychological findings

Recent research using a variety of modern neuroimaging techniques such as functional MRI has identified a number of important circuits for the generation of emotion and its regulation. Disruptions in these networks both structurally and functionally are thought to underpin mood disorders, and in bipolar disorder a number of findings are beginning to be replicated. For instance, anatomical and functional studies have identified differences in a number of brain regions in bipolar patients that include structures such as the prefrontal cortex, anterior cingulate and amygdala. However, these findings must still be viewed as tentative because most studies to date have involved relatively small numbers of subjects and the changes are not wholly consistent. In part this probably reflects the diversity of techniques that have been used to investigate bipolar disorder, but it may also highlight some intrinsic illness heterogeneity.

Clinically, these same brain regions, along with others such as the hippocampus, have been repeatedly implicated in the etiology of bipolar disorder. For example, neuropsychological studies that have attempted to profile the executive and mnemonic functions of patients with bipolar disorder have often found deficits in attention and memory that engage neural networks connecting prefrontal and subcortical brain regions. Of note the subtle neurocognitive compromise observed in patients with bipolar disorder does not appear to be limited to periods of acute illness. It would appear that even when seemingly well (i.e. euthymic), neuropsychological tests on bipolar patients reveal subtle neurocognitive deficits that potentially reflect a trait deficit. Whether these changes are indeed trait or state-related is not known. Further, the timing and extent to which such changes can be detected early in the course of bipolar disorder is yet to be determined. In fact it is not even clear whether these findings are unique to bipolar disorder. However, these findings do reflect the cognitive compromise that patients often report and are therefore important to acknowledge and better understand.

4.5 Conclusion

A comprehensive neurobiological explanation for bipolar disorder has not been achieved. However, there are many promising findings that demonstrate that the illness has a strong genetic basis and that environmental factors, possibly via the neuroendocrine 'stress axis', play a significant role.

References and further reading

Escamilla MA, Zavala JM (2008). Genetics of bipolar disorder. *Dialogues in Clinical Neuroscience*, **10**(2),129–39.

Newberg AR, Catapano LA, Zarate CA, Manji HK (2008). Neurobiology of bipolar disorder. *Expert Review of Neurotherapeutics*, **8**(1), 93–110.

Martinowich K, Schloesser RJ, Manji HK (2009). Bipolar disorder: from genes to behavior pathways. *The Journal of Clinical Investigation*, **119**(4), 726–36.

Kato T (2008). Moelcular neurobiology of bipolar disorder: a disease of 'mood stabilizing neurons'? *Trends in Neurosciences*, **31**(10), 495–503.

Pharmacotherapy for bipolar disorder

> **Key points**
> - All patients must have a baseline assessment that includes full medical history and laboratory evaluation prior to commencement of pharmacotherapy
> - The efficacy and safety profile varies between various anticonvulsants
> - There are clear differences in adverse event profiles between various atypical antipsychotics
> - Antidepressants should not be used in monotherapy for acute bipolar depression; there is no evidence for the efficacy of antidepressants in the long term treatment of bipolar depression.

5.1 Baseline assessment

Pharmacotherapy is the cornerstone of management of bipolar disorder. All patients should have a baseline assessment that includes medical history and laboratory investigations as outlined in Table 5.1 before commencing pharmacotherapy. This may not be possible in those that are acutely manic before emergency pharmacotherapy is prescribed, but in such situations the assessment should be completed as soon as the patient is able to co-operate.

5.2 Lithium

5.2.1 Efficacy

Lithium is effective for acute mania and for preventing both manic and depressive episodes of bipolar disorder. It is most effective in euphoric grandiose mania but less effective in those with dysphoric mania, comorbid substance abuse, and mania secondary to a neurological condition. The long term treatment with lithium reduces suicidal behaviour and suicide. Lithium is also effective in treating acute bipolar depression when dosed adequately.

Table 5.1 Baseline assessment for patients with bipolar disorder prior to pharmacotherapy (based on data from Ng et al., 2009)

	Recommendations
History	Medical history
	Substance abuse, cigarette smoking status and alcohol intake
	Family history of cardiovascular and cerebrovascular disease, hypertension, dyslipidaemia and diabetes mellitus
	Pregnancy and contraception (for women of childbearing age)
Examination	Physical examination if clinically indicated
	Waist circumference and/or BMI (weight [kg]/height [m]^2)
	Blood pressure
Investigations	Full blood count
	Drug screen
	Electrolytes, urea, creatinine
	Liver function tests
	Fasting blood glucose
	Fasting lipid profile
	Pregnancy test (if clinically indicated)

5.2.2 Baseline assessment

Thyroid stimulating hormone (TSH), serum calcium and an electro-cardiogram in those over the age of 40 should be performed in addition to the routine baseline investigations outlined in Table 5.1 in patients being commenced on lithium.

5.2.3 Dosing and monitoring

Lithium is well absorbed with a bioavailability close to 100%, not protein bound, eliminated renally unchanged, and has a half life of about 24 hours. In physically healthy subjects, lithium can be commenced at 900 mg to 1200 mg/day, usually given as a single dose at bedtime, and serum levels assessed at steady state (i.e. five days later and 12 hours after the last dose). The dose should be adjusted as clinically indicated to achieve serum lithium levels between 0.8–1.2 mmol/L as lower levels are less effective particularly for acute mania and acute bipolar depression. Serum levels should be measured at 6 month intervals and at ad-hoc if non-adherence or toxicity is suspected. Urea, creatinine, TSH and calcium should be measured at six month intervals during lithium therapy.

Lithium has a narrow therapeutic window and levels ≥1.5 mmol/L can be toxic and life threatening. Patients should be educated about adequate hydration and potential drug interactions particularly with over the counter medications, and advised to seek help immediately if any symptoms of toxicity such as confusion, coarse tremor, ataxia, lethargy, etc. appear.

5.2.4 Drug interactions

In most patients, lithium can be safely combined with other psychotropic medications such as antipsychotics, antidepressants and anticonvulsants. Thiazide diuretics, some NSAIDs such as diclofenac, indomethacin, ketoprofen, COX-2 inhibitors (celecoxib and rofecoxib), angiotensin I converting enzyme inhibitors (captopril, enalapril, fosinopril, lisinopril, perindopril), angiotensin II receptor type –I antagonists (candesartan, losartan, valsartan), renal disease, advanced age and dehydration increase serum lithium levels.

5.2.5 Common adverse events

The adverse events commonly associated with lithium and their management is listed in Table 5.2.

Table 5.2 Treatment of common adverse effects of lithium and anticonvulsants		
Medication	Adverse effect	Management options
Lithium, valproate, carbamazepine, lamotrigine	General	Decrease/divide dose. Change mood stabilizer.
Lithium, valproate, carabamazpine, lamotrigine	Gastrointestinal	Give with food. Change to extended release if nausea or vomiting. Change to suspension or immediate release if diarrhea. Symptomatic relief with gastrointestinal agents.
Lithium, valproate	Weight gain	Prior warning; diet; exercise Assess thyroid function. Add topiramate, zonisamide, or atomoxetine.
Lithium, carbamazepine	Neurotoxicity	Dose at bedtime. Gradual initiation to improve tolerance (with Li and carbamazepine).
Lithium, valproate	Tremor	Add propranolol; atenolol; pindolol.
Lithium, valproate	Hair loss	Add selenium 25–100 mcg/day, zinc 10–50 mg/day.
Lithium	Polyuria and polydipsia	Single bed time daily dose Add amiloride or thiazide diuretic.

Table 5.2 (Contd.)

Medication	Adverse effect	Management options
Lithium	Hypothyroidism	Thyroid replacement or change to a different mood stabilizer.
Valproate, carbamazepine	Hepatic	Discontinue carbamazepine/ valproate if hepatic indices > 3 x upper limit of normal.
Lamotrigine, carbamazepine	Rash	Gradual initiation. Limit other new antigens during initiation. Dermatology consultation regarding desensitization. Discontinue carbamazepine, lamotrigine if another explanation for rash is not evident.
Carbamazepine	Leukopenia, Blood dyscrasias	Add lithium. Discontinue carbamazepine if WBC < 3000 or neutrophils < 1000.
Valproate	Thrombocytopeania	Reduce the dose or switch to a different agent.
Carbamazepine	Hyponatremia	Decrease dose, dietary sodium supplementation, add lithium, demeclocycline, doxycycline.
Valproate	Polycystic ovary syndrome	Assessment and consultation, Hormonal therapy or switch to a different agent.
Lithium	Acne	Dermatological consultation, topical or systemic antibiotics.
Lithium	Lethargy, cognitive dulling	Reduce dose if possible, assess thyroid status.

5.3 Anticonvulsants (divalproex, carbamazepine, lamotrigine)

5.3.1 Efficacy

Divalproex (Depakote®, referred to as semisodium valproate in the UK) is effective in acute mania and in those with mixed episodes. Recent small controlled trials suggest that it has efficacy in treating acute bipolar depressive symptoms. Although the only maintenance placebo controlled trial failed, other controlled and open data as well as clinical experience supports the efficacy in maintenance treatment, but it does not appear to have an anti-suicidal effect like lithium.

Carbamazepine is effective in acute mania and it likely has efficacy in preventing both manic and depressive episodes. It may be particularly effective in non-classical bipolar disorder or those with comorbid neurological problems. Carbamazepine also has mild to moderate acute antidepressant properties.

Lamotrigine is ineffective in treating acute mania and should not be used for this purpose. It has mild to moderate acute antidepressant properties and thus is useful in treating acute bipolar depression. Lamotrigine has proven efficacy in prevention of bipolar depression but minimal efficacy in preventing manic episodes.

5.3.2 Baseline assessment

Assess for history of haematological or hepatic diseases and dermatological conditions including skin rashes prior to carbamazepine therapy. Those considered for valproate should have hepatic and menstrual status assessed routinely while those being considered for lamotrigine therapy should be assessed for allergic skin rashes including Steven Johnson syndrome or toxic epidermal necrolysis.

5.3.3 Dosing and monitoring

Valproate is available as valproic acid, divalproex (semisodium valproate in the UK) and divalproex extended release. It is well absorbed and has a bioavailability close to 100%. It is extensively metabolized and has an elimination half life of about 12 hours. Valproate can be started at 750 to 1,500 mg/day or 10–25 mg/kg/day and the dose can be titrated as tolerated to achieve target serum levels between 50–125 mcg/mL. Those with acute mania may need serum levels in the higher target range. Serum levels, blood counts, and liver function tests should be assessed at 6 month intervals and as clinically indicated. History of menstrual irregularities should be inquired for at each visit and further investigations such as ultrasound may be performed if polycystic ovary syndrome is suspected.

Carbamazepine has erratic absorption with a bioavailability of about 80%. It is extensively metabolized with a half life of 24 hours before auto-induction which decreases to about 8 hours following auto-induction. Carbamazepine is started at 200 mg twice a day, and the dose adjusted every one to four days as tolerated to a target dose between 600 mg to 1600 mg/day. The dose may require adjustment after 2 to 4 weeks as serum levels drop due to auto-induction. The target serum levels are 6–12 mcg/mL but no clear relationship has been demonstrated between serum levels and therapeutic efficacy. Patients with acute mania require more aggressive titration and likely higher doses for response. Blood counts and LFT's should be monitored at six month intervals.

Lamotrigine is absorbed well and is extensively metabolized with a half life of about 28 hours. The incidence of rash can be reduced by

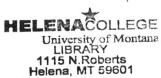

slow titration of lamotrigine with a starting dose of 25 mg/day for two weeks and increasing to 50 mg/day for another two weeks. Further increases can be made at 50 mg every week until target dose of 200 mg/day is reached. Some patients respond to lower doses while others may need higher doses up to 400 mg/day. The risk of rash is higher when lamotrigine is co-administered with valproate and hence the dose titration should be halved for those on concurrent valproate therapy as valproate doubles serum levels of lamotrigine. Conversely, the dose should be doubled for those on carbamazepine as carbamazepine halves serum levels of lamotrigine. Clinical experience suggests that breakthrough depressions often respond to dose increments of 25–50 mg. No relationship has been reported between serum levels and therapeutic efficacy. Patients should be warned of risk of skin rash and advised to report immediately if any skin rashes appear. If the skin rash is present in mucous membranes or becomes generalized and associated with fever, patients should be asked to stop lamotrigine and seek medical help urgently.

5.3.4 Drug interactions

Anticonvulsants can be safely combined with lithium. They can also be combined with each other but clinicians must be aware of pharmacokinetic interactions between various anticonvulsants so that dose adjustments and monitoring are done appropriately. For instance, valproate doubles serum levels of lamotrigine and increases levels of epoxide metabolite of carbamazepine while levels of valproate levels are significantly reduced by carbamazepine. Further, carbamazepine is an inducer of hepatic microsomal enzymes and induces metabolism of many commonly used psychotropic medications such as lamotrigine, risperidone, olanzapine, quetiapine, bupropion, sertraline, and many non-psychotropic medications such as warfarin and oral contraceptives etc. Thus, clinicians should be very vigilant and take special care in prescribing carbamazepine to bipolar patients who are taking other medications. Lamotrigine levels may be significantly reduced by oral contraceptives and lamotrigine may decrease the efficacy of oral contraceptives.

5.3.5 Common adverse events

The common adverse events of anticonvulsants and their management are listed in Table 5.2.

5.4 Newer anticonvulsants

Oxcarbazepine may be useful for treatment of acute mania but topiramate and gabapentin appear to be ineffective. Pregabalin and gabapentin are effective for treating anxiety and may be useful in treating co-morbid anxiety symptoms in bipolar disorder. Topiramate reduces appetite and causes weight loss and thus may have utility in treating weight gain associated with psychotropic medication use in bipolar disorder. No controlled trials exist to support the use of other anticonvulsants such as levatiracetam, felbamate, tiagabine and zonisamide in bipolar disorder.

CHAPTER 5 Pharmacotherapy for bipolar disorder

5.5 Conventional antipsychotics

Of the several conventional antipsychotics, chlorpromazpine and haloperidol are the most studied and both are effective in treating acute mania. Of these, haloperidol is the most commonly used as it is available in both the injectable and oral form. The dose ranges from 5 to 20 mg/day for acute mania and 0.2 mg/kg for the injectable preparation to reduce agitation. Zuclopenithixol acetate (Clopixol Acuphase®) 50 mg to 150 mg IM is also used to treat acute agitation and improve sleep as the effects may last up to two to three days after which patients may be switched to oral therapy with atypical antipsychotics. Apart from the risk of extrapyramidal symptoms, continuation of conventional antipsychotics is also associated with increased risk of depressive symptoms/episodes and tardive dyskinesia and thus longer term use of conventional agents is not recommended for bipolar patients.

5.6 Atypical antipsychotics

5.6.1 Efficacy

Evidence from controlled trials for the efficacy of atypical antipsychotics for various phases of bipolar disorder is summarized in Table 5.3. Although clozapine has not been assessed in placebo controlled trials, open randomized studies and clinical experience supports the efficacy in refractory acute mania and in long term treatment of refractory bipolar disorder.

Adjunctive risperidone, olanzapine, quetiapine and aripiprazole therapy to lithium or valproate is superior to monotherapy with lithium or valproate in acute mania. Adjunctive therapy particularly with quetiapine and possibly with risperidone, ziprasidone (not yet approved in UK) and olanzapine appear to provide additional benefit in long-term treatment of bipolar disorder.

5.6.2 Baseline assessment

Routine baseline assessment outlined above for all bipolar patients is sufficient and no additional tests are necessary prior to commencing atypical antipsychotics.

5.6.3 Dosages and monitoring

The doses of atypical antipsychotics are listed in Table 5.4. There is no evidence for relationship between serum levels and efficacy and hence assessment of serum levels is not necessary for therapeutic purposes. There are specific local requirements for monitoring those on clozapine such as weekly or biweekly blood counts and these should be adhered to. In addition, all patients on atypical antipsychotics should have their weight assessed monthly in the first three months, and every third month thereafter. In addition, fasting glucose and lipid profile should be assessed at three and six months and every six to 12 months thereafter for the duration of therapy.

Table 5.3 Atypical antipsychotics in bipolar disorder: efficacy summary

	Acute treatment		Maintenance/ continuation treatment	
	Mania	Depression	Mania	Depression
Olanzapine	++	+	++	+
Risperidone	++	?	++	+?
Quetiapine	++	++	++	++
Ziprasidone	++	?	+ (as adjunct)	?
Aripiprazole	++	–	+	–
Asenapine (not licensed in UK)	++	?	?	?
Paliperidone	++	?	?	?

++ = at least one good randomized controlled trial (RCT) showing clinically significant effects; + = at least one RCT showing some effect; – = RCT evidence of a lack of clinically significant effects; ? = uncertain or no controlled data available.

Table 5.4 Atypical antipsychotics: dosing and adverse events

Drug (range , mg/day)	½ life	Wt gain	Glucose + lipids	Cardiac effects	Pro-lactin	EPS	Sedation
Quetiapine (150–800)	6	++	++	–	O	O	++
Risperidone (2–6)	6–24	+	+	–	++	++	+
Olanzapine (5–20)	30	+++	+++	–	+	+	++
Ziprasidone (40–160)	7	O	O	QT prolongation	O	+	O
Aripiprazole (10–30)	72	O	O	–	O	+	O
Paliperidone (6–12)	23	+	+	–	+	++	+

O = none; + = minimal/rare; ++mild/occasional; +++=moderate/frequent.

5.6.4 Drug interactions

Serum levels of clozapine and olanzapine are significantly increased by fluoxamine and possibly fluoxetine while carbamazepine reduces levels of clozapine, olanzapine, risperidone, quetiapine and aripiprazole.

5.6.5 Common adverse events

Table 5.4 lists common side effects and rates the propensity of each atypical to cause these. In addition, somnolence, dizziness, dry mouth, constipation and asthenia are common with olanzapine and quetiapine while akathisia and agitation are not uncommon with ziprasidone and aripiprazole. Aripiprazole may also cause gastrointestinal adverse effects such as nausea, dyspepsia, vomiting and diarrhea. Clozapine causes agranulocytosis which can be life threatening and hence those on clozapine should follow local monitoring guidelines. Clozapine should not be combined with carbamazepine due to increased risk of agranulocytosis. Clozapine also causes sialorrhea commonly which is a nuisance for many patients. Prolongation of QTc interval is of concern with ziprasidone.

5.7 Antidepressants

5.7.1 Efficacy

Despite the widely held belief that antidepressants are effective, few placebo controlled trials assessed their efficacy for bipolar depression. Antidepressant monotherapy is not recommended for bipolar depression due to concerns about a manic switch and destabilization of the course of bipolar disorder. In particular, tricyclic antidepressants are not recommended for bipolar depression as they have greater propensity to switch patients into mania and induce rapid cycling. Although there are some negative studies, adjunctive therapy of modern antidepressants was shown to be effective in acute bipolar depression in a meta-analysis and experience of some clinicians is consistent with this. However, there is little evidence for efficacy or safety of antidepressants in long term treatment of bipolar depression. If adjunctive antidepressants are used for acute bipolar depression, they should be tapered and discontinued within 8 weeks of remission of depression.

Bupropion and serotonergic antidepressants are commonly used as adjunctive therapy. Among the modern antidepressants, venlafaxine appears to have greater propensity for causing a manic switch.

5.7.2 Baseline assessment

No additional investigations are required prior to commencing antidepressant adjunctive therapy.

5.7.3 Dosages and monitoring

Fluoxetine, paroxetine and citalopram are dosed between 20–60 mg/day while fluvoxamine and sertraline are dosed between 100–300 and 100–200 mg/day, respectively. Bupropion is given at 200–450 mg/day, escitalopram at 10–30 mg/day, duloxetine at 40–80 mg/day, and venlafaxine 75–300 mg/day. Patients should be informed about the potential risk of a manic/hypomanic switch. Although no studies have reported an increase in suicidal ideation with antidepressants in bipolar depressed patients, it is prudent clinical practice to assess for suicidal ideation in all bipolar depressed patients at each clinical visit. Sexual dysfunction with serotonergic antidepressants is a common reason for treatment non-adherence and this should be addressed at each clinical visit.

5.7.4 Drug interactions

Antidepressants are metabolized by CYP450 isoenzymes. Fluoxetine and paroxetine are metabolized by CYP2D6. Both these potently inhibit CYP2D6 while sertraline and bupropion moderately inhibit this enzyme, thus potentially increasing the levels of other drugs metabolized by CYP2D6 such as tricyclics and risperidone, etc. CYP3A3/4 metabolizes sertraline and citalopram while fluoxetine and fluvoxamine inhibit CYP3A3/4. Fluvoxamine in addition can inhibit CYP1A2 and increase levels of clozapine, warfarin, etc.

5.7.5 Common adverse events

These include gastrointestinal (nausea, vomiting, and diarrhea), central nervous system (drowsiness, headache, tremor, agitation, sleep disturbance), dry mouth, and sexual side effects. Fluvoxamine causes the most GI distress while weight gain is not uncommon with paroxetine. Venlafaxine and duloxetine cause less sexual dysfunction than SSRIs. Changes in blood pressure and withdrawal symptoms are common with venlafaxine. Paroxetine also causes significant withdrawal symptoms. Bupropion does not cause sexual side effects but at higher doses, there is an increased risk of seizures. Bupropion should not be prescribed for those with co-morbid eating disorders or for those with other risk factors for seizures.

References and further reading

Gijsman HJ, Geddes JR, Rendell JM, Nolen WA, and Goodwin GM (2004). Antidepressants for bipolar depression: A systematic review of randomized, controlled trials. *Am J Psychiatry,* **161**(9), 1537–47.

Ketter TA, Wang PW (2009). Psychotropic Medications in bipolar disorder: Pharmacodynamics, pharmacokinetics, drug interactions, adverse effects and their management. In Yatham LN, Kusumakar V (eds), *Bipolar Disorder: A Guide to Clinical Management,* 437–550.

Murray M (2006) Role of CYP pharmacogenetics and drug-drug interactions in the efficacy and safety of atypical and other antipsychotic agents. *J Pharm Pharmacol*, **58**(7), 871–85.

Yatham LN, Kusumakar V (2009). Anticonvulsants in the treatment of bipolar disorder: A review of efficacy. In Yatham LN, Kusumakar V (eds), *Bipolar Disorder: A Guide to Clinical Management*, 381–410.

Chapter 6

Psychological treatments

> **Key points**
> - Psychological treatments are used mainly as adjuncts to pharmacotherapy
> - Psychoeducation, interpersonal and social rhythm therapy (IPSRT), family focussed therapy (FFT), and cognitive behavioural therapy (CBT) are all effective as adjunctive treatment in preventing relapse of mood episodes
> - Psychoeducation is cheap and effective and should be offered to all patients with bipolar disorder
> - Because of cost, CBT, FFT and IPSRT should be offered only when they are clearly indicated or to those who have not responded to pharmacotherapy and psychoeducation.

6.1 Introduction

Pharmacotherapy is the foundation of treatment in bipolar disorder. Psychological treatments are not used alone but rather as adjuncts to medications to improve outcomes through enhancing treatment adherence, coping skills and illness management. All forms of psychosocial treatments in BD involve some elements of psychoeducation.

6.2 Types of psychological treatments

6.2.1 Psychoeducation

6.2.1.1 *Overview*

The main objective of psychoeducation is to empower patients to manage their illness effectively. This is achieved by helping patients to become aware of symptoms, course and treatment of the disorder, improve treatment adherence, recognize early warning signs of relapse, avoid potential triggers of the episodes such as substance abuse, learn coping strategies, and promote regular sleep wake cycles and social activities.

Psychoeducation can be provided in an individual or group format. The latter is more popular and more cost effective. Group is psychoeducation is offered to a group of patients with bipolar disorder or a group consisting of four to six bipolar patients and their family members or a group consisting of just caregivers. The number of sessions in the group varies and can range from as few as five sessions to as many as 21 or more.

6.2.1.2 *Efficacy*

There is good evidence that adjunctive psychoeducation is effective in reducing relapse rates in euthymic bipolar patients. Time to relapse of a mood episode and time to relapse of a manic episode are significantly longer in those that receive psychoeducation compared with those that receive treatment as usual. The benefits are apparent for up to five years with some booster sessions. Multifamily psycho-education groups are beneficial for bipolar patients with dysfunctional families with high expressed emotion. Group psychoeducation for caregivers has also been shown to improve outcomes for bipolar patients.

6.2.2 Cognitive behavioural therapy (CBT)

6.2.2.1 *Overview*

The CBT as described in the published manuals for bipolar disorder combines cognitive and behavioural tools with psychoeducation. Cognitive component of the CBT is used to help patients identify automatic dysfunctional thoughts (catastrophizing, minimization or maximization, negative inference, overgeneralization, etc.) and under-lying assumptions and change those by rationally challenging them. An active Socratic questioning style is used during the sessions to train patients to substitute rational thoughts. Other components of CBT facilitate patients to learn about illness management which include recognition of early warning signs, medication adherence, and coping strategies. CBT is offered over a course of 20 to 50 sessions with some booster sessions over the course of the following few months.

6.2.2.2 *Efficacy*

CBT was assessed for efficacy in acute bipolar depression and in prevention of relapse of mood episodes in bipolar disorder. In a large Systematic Treatment Enhancement Program for bipolar disorder (STEP-BD) trial, time to recovery from acute bipolar depression and response rates were similar in the CBT, IPSRT and FFT groups and significantly greater compared with those that were assigned to the collaborative care group.

In euthymic bipolar 1 patients, CBT was effective in reducing relapse rates, days in episodes and hospitalization during the 12 month study period but during the 18 month follow up period, no differences emerged between the CBT and the treatment as usual groups, although original difference in time to relapse between the groups persisted. CBT was no more effective than group psychoeducation in reducing the morbidity or time to recovery or relapse in a large Canadian Trial. Further, in the trial conducted in the United Kingdom, CBT was no more effective than treatment as usual in preventing a recurrence of a new episode when it was offered to a broader group of symptomatic and asymptomatic bipolar patients and those with comorbidity. In this study, the benefit was apparent only for those patients who had fewer (<12) prior mood episodes.

In summary, CBT appears to be beneficial for only a select subgroup of bipolar patients.

6.2.3 Interpersonal and Social Rhythm Therapy (IPSRT)

6.2.3.1 Overview
IPSRT integrates the principles of the interpersonal therapy (IPT) and theories of biology of circadian rhythms. The IPSRT combines psychoeducation (focus on learning about bipolar disorder and its impact, medication management including efficacy and side effects, and learning about early warning signs of relapse), social rhythm therapy (using a five item social rhythm metric to establish social rhythms and their impact on mood and promoting social rhythm stability through life changes) and IPT (addressing interpersonal issues such as unresolved grief, role disputes, role transition, or interpersonal deficits/social isolation as well as grief for the lost healthy self) as strategies to address interpersonal difficulties, enhance medication adherence and minimize the impact of life events on social rhythms with the objective to promote circadian integrity and thus minimize risk of recurrence of mood episodes.

6.2.3.2 *Efficacy*
In acute trials, patients receiving IPSRT had greater social rhythm stability and shorter median time to remission (patients with index depressive episode) compared with those receiving intensive clinical management (ICM). As well, patients who received IPSRT during the acute phase survived longer without relapse/recurrence in a two year study compared with those who received ICM during the acute phase. The recovery rates were higher in the STEP-BD trial in bipolar patients assigned to IPSRT compared with those that received collaborative care.

6.2.4 Family Focused Treatment (FFT)

6.2.4.1 *Overview*
FFT was developed partly based on the expressed emotions (EE) literature which showed that relapse rates were higher amongst BD patients in families with high EE. The FFT is offered to the patient and family members as an integrated treatment over a nine month period in 21 sessions over 3 stages. These include a psychoeducation stage

(information about symptoms, course, diagnosis and management offered in didactic format), a communication enhancement training stage (promoting active listening, expression of positive feelings, constructive negative feedback and making positive requests for changes in behaviours), and a problem solving skills training (facilitating identification of problems, generating and evaluating solutions and implementing them) stage.

6.2.4.2 *Efficacy*
Controlled trials suggest that patients who receive FFT have longer periods of mood stability and lower rates of relapse compared to those that receive crisis management or collaborative care. The FFT is at least as effective as other forms of intensive therapy.

6.3 When psychotherapy and for what phases?

6.3.1 Acute mania
Many manic patients have little insight and are often not amenable for any form of therapy. Hence, it is not surprising that no systematic data are available for the efficacy of adjunctive psychological treatments in mania. However, as manic symptoms improve, psychoeducation could be commenced and can be offered initially in an individual format and later in a group format as appropriate.

6.3.2 Acute bipolar depression
The STEP-BD data suggest that the time to recovery is shorter and response rates are greater in bipolar depressed patients who receive any form of psychotherapy (CBT, IPSRT, or FFT) compared with those that receive collaborative care. However, the cost of these treatments can be substantial and hence these perhaps should be offered only to those that are non-responsive to standard pharmacotherapy and psychoeducation.

6.3.3 Maintenance treatment of bipolar disorder
Given that group psychoeducation has shown similar efficacy to CBT and is relatively cheap, this should be offered to all patients with bipolar disorder to reduce the risk of relapse in conjunction with pharmacotherapy. Those that relapse despite adequate pharmacotherapy and psychoeducation should be offered other forms of therapy. The FFT should be considered for bipolar patients with family or marital conflicts and those from dysfunctional families with high expressed emotions. CBT may be considered for bipolar patients with fewer prior mood episodes but it has efficacy mainly in those who were euthymic at the time of commencement of therapy. The IPSRT appears to work the best when it is offered from the acute

symptomatic phase. Overall, the evidence suggests that psychoeducation, CBT, IPSRT, and FTT are effective in reducing relapse rates and prolonging time to relapse when used as adjuncts to pharmacotherapy. Given the efficacy from controlled trials for adjunctive psychosocial treatments, psychoeducation for all bipolar patients and FFT, IPSRT or CBT to those that are non responsive to psychoeducation should be offered to improve outcomes.

References and further reading

Colom F, Vieta E, Martinez-Aran A, Reinares M, Goikolea JM, Benabarre A et al. (2003a). A randomized trial on the efficacy of group psychoeducation in the prophylaxis of recurrences in bipolar patients whose disease is in remission. *Archives of General Psychiatry*, **60**(4), 402–7.

Frank E, Kupfer DJ, Thase ME et al. (2005). Two-year outcomes for interpersonal and social rhythm therapy in individuals with bipolar I disorder. *Archives of General Psychiatry*, **62**(9), 996–1004.

Lam DH, Watkins ER, Hayward P et al. (2003). A randomized controlled study of cognitive therapy for relapse prevention for bipolar affective disorder: Outcome for the first year. *Archives of General Psychiatry*, **60**(2), 145–52.

Miklowitz DJ, Otto MW, Frank E, et al. (2007). Psychosocial treatments for bipolar depression: A 1-year randomized trial from the Systematic Treatment Enhancement Program. *Archives of General Psychiatry*, **64**(4), 419–27.

Reinares M, Colom F, Sanchez-Moreno J et al. (2008). Impact of caregiver group psychoeducation on the course and outcome of bipolar patients in remission: a randomised controlled trial. *Bipolar Disorders*, **10**(4), 511–19.

Scott J, Paykel E, Morriss R et al. (2006). Cognitive-behavioural therapy for severe and recurrent bipolar disorders: A randomized controlled trial. *British Journal of Psychiatry*, **188**, 313–20.

Chapter 7

Treatment guidelines for management of bipolar disorder

Key points

- First line treatments for mania include monotherapy with lithium or valproate or an atypical antipsychotic or a combination of lithium or valproate plus an atypical antipsychotic
- If antidepressants are used in conjunction with a mood stabilizer for acute bipolar depression, they should be tapered and discontinued within eight weeks of remission
- Lamotrigine, quetiapine and lithium are effective in preventing a depressive relapse
- Lithium, valproate, and all atypical antipsychotics assessed to date appear to have efficacy in preventing mania.

7.1 Introduction

Several guidelines exist for management of bipolar disorder. The management strategies outlined in this chapter are based on the Canadian Network for Mood and Anxiety Treatments (CANMAT) guidelines which take into account the evidence for efficacy and adverse events in formulating first, second and third line treatments for managing patients with bipolar disorder.

7.1 Acute mania

Recommendations for treatment of acute mania based on the efficacy and adverse event profile are listed in Table 7.1 and the treatment algorithm is outlined in Figure 7.1.

7.1.1 Emergency management

All patients with acute mania should be assessed for risk of aggressive behaviour/violence and steps must be taken to ensure safety for the patient and the treatment team. This may include physical restraint, placement of the patient in a quiet room, and administering atypical antipsychotics, benzodiazepines or conventional antipsychotic medications to control agitation rapidly. The choice of medication should be based on previous history of response and tolerability. When possible, oral atypical antipsychotics should be offered first but if the patient refuses, injectable olanzapine, ziprasidone or aripiprazole should be considered. First generation antipsychotics such as injectable loxapine or haloperidol or zuclopenthixol are also effective and could be combined with benzodiazepines for synergistic effect and to reduce the risk of dystonic reactions. The switch to oral atypical antipsychotic and/or mood stabilizer therapy should be made as soon as the patient has regained some insight and willing to accept oral medications.

Table 7.1 Recommendations for pharmacological treatment of acute mania

First line	Lithium, divalproex (semisodium valproate (Depakote®) in the UK), olanzapine, risperidone, quetiapine, aripiprazole, ziprasidone (not yet approved in UK), lithium or divalproex + risperidone, lithium or divalproex + quetiapine, lithium or divalproex + olanzapine, lithium or divalproex + aripiprazole
Second line	Carbamazepine, ECT, lithium + divalproex, asenapine, lithium or divalproex + asenapine (not licensed in UK), paliperidone monotherapy
Third line	Haloperidol, chlorpromazine, lithium or divalproex + haloperidol, lithium + carbamazepine, clozapine, oxcarbazepine, tamoxifen
Not recommended	Monotherapy with gabapentin, topiramate, lamotrigine, verapamil, tiagabine, risperidone + carbamazepine, olanzapine + carbamazepine

ECT = electroconvulsive therapy.

Figure 7.1 Treatment algorithm for acute mania

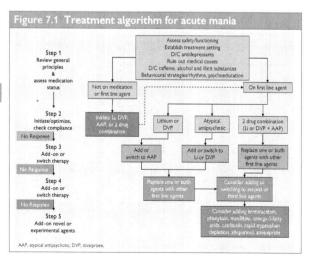

AAP, atypical antipsychotic; DVP, divalproex.

48

7.1.2 First-line treatments

Overall, there does not appear to be any significant difference in efficacy or response rates between monotherapy with lithium, valproate, or various atypical antipsychotics. Approximately 40% to 50% of patients with acute mania respond to monotherapy within three weeks, and response rates are about 20% greater with a combination of lithium or valproate and an atypical antipsychotic. Although carbamazepine and haloperidol are effective, these are not considered first line because of their propensity for drug interactions and adverse event profile.

Whether an acute manic patient be treated with monotherapy or combination therapy and with which medication or combination of medications should be based on symptom profile of a patient, need for rapid behavioural control, previous history of response and the acceptability of adverse event profile of medications. Those with euphoric/grandiose mania respond well to lithium monotherapy but patients with mixed states often respond better to valproate or an atypical antipsychotic or the combination. Although evidence is lacking, clinical experience suggests that patients with psychotic mania or those with severe mania may be more rapidly controlled with a combination treatment.

7.1.3 When to switch or add?

If symptoms have not improved by at least 20% with optimal therapeutic doses within two weeks as measured by changes in rating scale scores such as Young Mania Rating Scale or as determined by clinical impression, the clinician should consider switching a patient from lithium or valproate to an atypical antipsychotic or vice versa. If there was some improvement in symptoms but further progress is slower, increasing the dose of medications to maximum tolerable limits should be considered before adding a second medication. If a patient was on a combination and response is less than 20% by the end of the second week, one of the medications should be switched as indicated in Figure 7.1.

7.1.4 Second-line treatments

Although new atypical antipsychotics such as paliperidone and asenapine have shown efficacy, these are listed as second line treatments because of lack of clinical experience and effectiveness data. Most manic patients will respond to mono or combination therapy of first line treatments. Hence, these should be tried first before second line options are considered.

7.1.5 Third-line treatments

In patients who do not respond fully or those that have idiosyncratic responses or tolerability problems with first or second line treatments, third line treatments may be tried. If conventional antipsychotics are used for treating mania, they should be discontinued within six to eight weeks of complete remission of mania as continuation increases the risk of depressive episodes in bipolar patients.

7.1.6 Psychosocial strategies

These should commence in conjunction with pharmacotherapy as soon as a patient becomes amenable. All patients should be offered psychoeducation (see Chapter 8 for details) and other therapies as appropriate. The goal should be to empower the patient to take responsibility for managing bipolar disorder effectively.

7.2 Acute bipolar depression

Pharmacological treatment options for bipolar depression are listed in Table 7.2 and treatment algorithm is outlined in Figure 7.2.

7.2.1 In-patient or out-patient treatment

Risk of self harm/suicide is greatest during bipolar depression and about 15% of bipolar patients commit suicide. Hence, suicide risk, severity of depression, and availability of psychosocial support are the major factors that determine whether a patient is treated on an in-patient or outpatient setting.

7.2.2 Psychosocial treatments

No controlled trials have assessed the efficacy of psychosocial treatments for acute bipolar depression in monotherapy. Hence, psychosocial strategies are predominantly used as adjunctive treatments to

Table 7.2 Recommendations for the pharmacological treatment of acute bipolar I depression[a]	
First line	Lithium, lamotrigine, quetiapine, lithium or divalproex + SSRI, olanzapine + SSRI, lithium + divalproex, lithium or divalproex + bupropion
Second line	Quetiapine + SSRI, divalproex, lithium or divalproex + lamotrigine, adjunctive modafinil
Third line	Carbamazepine, olanzapine, lithium + carbamazepine, lithium + pramipexole, lithium or divalproex + venlafaxine, lithium + MAOI, ECT, lithium or divalproex or AAP + TCA, lithium or divalproex or carbamazepine + SSRI + lamotrigine, adjunctive EPA, adjunctive riluzole, adjunctive topiramate
Not recommended	Gabapentin monotherapy, aripiprazole monotherapy

[a]The management of a bipolar depressive episode with antidepressants remains complex. The clinician must balance the desired effect of remission with the undesired effect of switching.

AAP, atypical antipsychotic; ECT, electroconvulsive therapy; EPA, eicosapentanoic acid; SSRI, selective serotonin reuptake inhibitor; ZIP, ziprasidone.

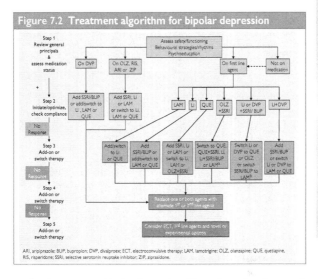

Figure 7.2 Treatment algorithm for bipolar depression

ARI, aripiprazole; BUP, bupropion; DVP, divalproex; ECT, electroconvulsive therapy; LAM, lamotrigine; OLZ, olanzapine; QUE, quetiapine; RIS, risperidone; SSRI, selective serotonin reuptake inhibitor; ZIP, ziprasidone.

medications to treat bipolar depression. Given that adjunctive cognitive behavioural therapy, interpersonal and social rhythm therapy as well as family focused treatment have been shown to be superior to collaborative care, they should be considered if resources are available, particularly for those with refractory bipolar depression.

7.2.3 First-line treatments

Patients with bipolar depression who are drug free should be commenced on lithium, quetiapine or lamotrigine monotherapy. For lithium to be effective, serum levels should be maintained at ≥0.8 mmol/l. A combination of lithium or valproate plus bupropion or serotonergic antidepressant is commonly used in clinical practice and may be appropriate for some bipolar depressed patients. Antidepressants should not be used in those with a history of rapid cycling or severe manias unless other first and second line treatments have been tried and found ineffective. Olanzapine plus serotonergic antidepressant combination is effective, and may be particularly appropriate for those with psychotic bipolar depression.

Patients who experience a breakthrough depressive episode while taking a first line treatment should be optimized (which might include ensuring that patient had been taking adequate doses for adequate period of time) before other options are considered. Those that relapse while taking valproate may also be optimized given the evidence for its efficacy from three small double blind placebo controlled trials. However, those that relapse while on an atypical antipsychotic other than quetiapine should be treated as outlined in Figure 7.2.

7.2.4 When to switch or add?

This issue has not been studied systematically. In general, if a patient has not improved by at least 20% within four weeks, addition of or switch to other medications should be considered. A shorter time frame and a more aggressive strategy might be appropriate in patients who are extremely distressed or suicidal. Small doses of atypical antipsychotics may be used to control acute distress or agitation.

7.2.5 Second-line treatments

In those with poor or inadequate response to two or more first line monotherapy strategies, combination of other first line treatments or first and second line treatment combinations might be appropriate. If lamotrigine is added to divalproex (semisodium valproate (Depakote®) in the UK), the dose titration of lamotrigine should be very slow in order to minimize the risk of skin rash and Steven Johnson syndrome and toxic epidermal necrolysis, both of which can be life threatening.

7.2.6 When to use electroconvulsive therapy (ECT)

Although controlled evidence is not available, open studies and clinical experience suggest that ECT is very effective and likely works faster than pharmacological treatments. Although ECT is recommended as a third line for acceptability reasons and side effects, it should be considered earlier for those with psychotic depression, those that are extremely distressed and suicidal, those that are not drinking and eating and thus pose medical risk, and those in the first trimester of pregnancy.

7.3 Maintenance treatment of bipolar disorder

7.3.1 Why and when maintenance treatment?

The majority (up to 80%) of patients with bipolar disorder relapse within five years of remission of an acute mood episode without maintenance treatment. Acute mood episodes are associated with significant impairment in functioning as well as personal and social negative consequences. Furthermore, patients with a history of multiple mood episodes have structural brain changes, greater impairment in cognitive and psychosocial functioning, are more likely to relapse and less likely to respond to acute and maintenance therapy. Therefore, it is important to offer maintenance treatment to all patients with bipolar disorder including those that had their first manic episode to prevent new mood episodes and the associated consequences.

7.3.2 What are the goals of maintenance?

The objectives should be to prevent recurrence/relapse of mood episodes, improve functioning as well as quality of life, and reduce the risk of suicide and suicide attempts. Sub-syndromal symptoms increase the risk of relapse and hence those should be aggressively treated.

7.3.3 Pharmacological treatment options for maintenance

Recommendations for maintenance treatment are listed in Table 7.3.

Several medications have been recommended as first line treatments. The clinician should consider the features listed in Table 7.4 in choosing the most appropriate option for a given patient. As a general rule, medication that worked for an acute episode is also likely to be effective in preventing relapse/recurrence of a mood episode, and hence use that first before considering other options. Quetiapine has similar magnitude of efficacy in preventing both manic and

Table 7.3 Recommendations for maintenance pharmacotherapy of bipolar disorder	
First line	Lithium, lamotrigine monotherapy (limited efficacy in preventing mania), divalproex, olanzapine, quetiapine, lithium or divalproex+ quetiapine, risperidone LAI, adjunctive risperidone LAI, aripiprazole (mainly for preventing mania), adjunctive ziprasidone
Second line	Carbamazepine, lithium + divalproex, lithium + carbamazepine, lithium or divalproex + olanzapine, lithium + risperidone, lithium + lamotrigine, olanzapine + fluoxetine
Third line	Adjunctive phenytoin, adjunctive clozapine, adjunctive ECT, adjunctive topiramate, adjunctive omega-3-fatty acids, adjunctive oxcarbazepine, or adjunctive gabapentin
Not recommended	Adjunctive flupentixol, monotherapy with gabapentin, topiramate or antidepressants

ECT=electroconvulsive therapy, LAI=long acting injection, SSRI=selective serotonin reuptake inhibitor.

Table 7.4 Issues to consider for maintenance treatment

1. Use for maintenance the same medication that worked for an acute episode
2. Consider predominant polarity
   a) Depressive polarity (More depressions than manias) – lamotrigine, quetiapine, lithium but not aripiprazole
   b) Manic polarity (more manias than depressions) – any first line except lamotrigine
   c) No polarity (manias and depressions occur in equal frequency) – quetiapine, lithium, valproate,
3. Past history of maintenance response
4. Family history of maintenance response
5. Consider combination maintenance if previous history of partial response to monotherapy.

depressive episodes while lithium, divalproex, and olanzapine have better efficacy in preventing mania than depression. Aripiprazole monotherapy should be used mainly for those with infrequent depressive episodes as it has minimal efficacy in preventing depressive relapses. In contrast, lamotrigine has greater efficacy in preventing depression and minimal efficacy in preventing manic episodes. Risperidone long acting injectable has shown promise in refractory bipolar disorder as an adjunctive therapy and the improved efficacy may be related to improved treatment adherence with this medication.

7.3.4 Breakthrough episodes/lack of efficacy

Treatment non-adherence is common in bipolar disorder. Hence, if a patient has a breakthrough episode while on maintenance treatment, treatment adherence should be assessed before switching to or adding on another medication. Patients who are partially responsive to monotherapy should be offered a combination therapy to treat sub-syndromal symptoms and thus reduce the risk of relapse. Risk of manic relapse can be significantly reduced by combining lithium or valproate with an atypical antipsychotic while risk of depressive relapse can be reduced by the addition of lamotrigine or quetiapine to lithium or valproate or by combining lamotrigine with an atypical antipsychotic. Antidepressants adjunctive therapy if used to treat sub-syndromal depressive symptoms should be tapered within eight weeks of full remission of depressive symptoms to minimize risk of manic switch.

7.3.5 Monitoring

Patients should be routinely asked at each visit about any difficulty taking medications and adverse events. If adverse events are not treated, patients will likely become non-adherent. If adverse events can not be resolved, alternative maintenance treatment options should be considered.

7.3.6 Role of psychological treatments

Adjunctive psychosocial treatments (see Chapter 6) reduce relapse rates. Hence, all patients should be offered either group or individual psychoeducation as a first option as this is likely cheaper than other psychosocial treatments. In patients who relapse, other adjunctive psychosocial treatments should be considered.

7.4 Rapid cycling bipolar disorder

7.4.1 General principles

Since acute mood episodes are shorter and often remit spontaneously, the focus of treatment in rapid cycling bipolar patients should be prevention of recurrence of mood episodes. This may include addressing factors that promote cycling and using medications to stabilize mood. Substance abuse, hypothyroidism or other endocrine problems should be promptly treated. Antidepressant medications should be avoided and antidepressants should be discontinued in those that are taking these medications.

7.4.2 Pharmacological management

Valproate and lithium are considered first line treatments for rapid cycling bipolar disorder based on a recent controlled trial which showed that the relapse rates were no different between the two treatments in patients who were stabilized with the combination of lithium and valproate. If monotherapy with either of these medications is ineffective, combination therapy is appropriate. Those with breakthrough depression should have lamotrigine or quetiapine added while those with breakthrough hypomania or mania could have an atypical antipsychotic added to prevent further recurrences. If a patient is refusing triple therapy or has difficulty tolerating adverse events, a clinical decision as to whether lithium or valproate was less effective for the patient should be made based on the information available and the less effective medication may be substituted with an atypical antipsychotic. Adding risperidone long acting injectable to treatment as usual has shown efficacy and this should be offered for those that continue to cycle with above strategies. Hypermetabolic doses of T4 or clozapine are useful in some patients. Psychosocial treatments as adjuncts are often helpful in improving outcome by improving treatment adherence and coping strategies.

7.5 Bipolar II disorder

Bipolar II disorder is common, often inadequately treated, and is associated with significant impairment in functioning and disability. Diagnosis is often missed as patients often do not report hypomanic episodes as they do not perceive these as problematic. However, behaviour during hypomanic episodes can result in significant financial, legal and psychosocial problems.

7.5.1 Pharmacological treatment

7.5.1.1 *Hypomania*

No controlled studies exist for hypomania but clinical experience suggests that all antimanic agents are effective in treating acute hypomanic symptoms. The significant challenge here might be convincing the patient to take medication as many may not perceive their behaviour as being problematic.

7.5.1.2 *Acute bipolar 2 depression*

Recommendations for acute bipolar 2 depression are outlined in Table 7.5. Patients who are drug free should be treated with quetiapine monotherapy as this medication has the best evidence. Monotherapy with lamotrigine, lithium, or divalproex (semisodium valproate (Depakote®) in the UK) are appropriate alternate options in those that do not respond to or refuse quetiapine. Bupropion and serotonergic antidepressants can be combined with lithium or valproate or an atypical antipsychotic as the risk of switch is lower in bipolar 2 patients compared with those with bipolar I disorder. Augmentation with pramipexole or modafinil may be required in some patients to relieve acute depressive symptoms. Antidepressant monotherapy may be considered in a very small subset of bipolar 2 patients with no previous history of mood switch, infrequent hypomanias and no family history of bipolar I disorder, but only after risks of switch have been carefully explained to the patients and family members.

7.5.1.3 *Maintenance treatment of bipolar 2 disorder*

Depressive symptoms and episodes outnumber hypomanic symptoms/episodes by a ratio of up to 37:1 in bipolar 2 patients. Hence the major objective should be to prevent relapse/recurrence of depressive symptoms without destabilizing the course of bipolar 2 disorder. Maintenance treatment often begins after resolution of an acute depressive episode. With the exception of antidepressant monotherapy, as a general rule, continue the same medication/s that worked for an acute episode. If monotherapy fails, combination of two first line treatments or a combination of an atypical antipsychotic or lithium or valproate plus bupropion or serotonergic antidepressant may be appropriate.

Table 7.5 Recommendations for pharmacological treatment of acute bipolar 2 depression	
First line	Quetiapine
Second line	Lithium, lamotrigine, divalproex, lithium or divalproex + antidepressants, lithium + divalproex, atypical antipsychotics + antidepressants
Third line	Antidepressant monotherapy (particularly for those with infrequent hypomanias), switch to alternate antidepressant, ziprasidone
Not recommended	See text on antidepressants for recommendations regarding antidepressant monotherapy

7.6 Bipolar spectrum disorders

Patients with bipolar spectrum disorders are common and yet virtually, no controlled trials exist for bipolar spectrum disorders.

7.6.1 Treatment

Treatment decisions should be made on a case by case basis. As a general rule, treatment should be offered if there is distress or dysfunction. Supportive therapy or other psychosocial options may be sufficient to relieve distress in some cases. If pharmacological treatment is offered, monitor symptom changes, adverse events and periodically review the progress and need for continued medication use.

References and further reading

Yatham LN, Kennedy SH, O'Donovan C et al. (2005). CANMAT Guidelines for management of patients with bipolar disorder: consensus and controversies. Bipolar Disorders, **7**(3), 5–69.

Yatham LN, Kennedy SH, O'Donovan C et al. (2007). CANMAT Guidelines for management of patients with bipolar disorder: an update for 2007. Bipolar Disorders, **8**(6), 721–39, 200.

Yatham LN, Kennedy SH, Schaffer A et al. (2009). Canadian Network for Mood and Anxiety Treatments (CANMAT) and International Society for Bipolar Disorders (ISBD) Collaborative Update of CANMAT Guidelines for the management of Patients with Bipolar Disorder: Update 2009. Bipolar Disorders, **11**(3), 225–55.

Chapter 8

Special populations

Key points

- Diagnosis of bipolar disorder in children is challenging; comprehensive assessment and prospective follow up may be necessary in some cases to make a definitive diagnosis
- First episode mania in elderly is uncommon; rule out organic causes before making a diagnosis of bipolar disorder in the elderly
- Few studies systematically assessed the efficacy of medications in children, elderly, pregnant and postpartum women with bipolar disorder; treatment decisions must carefully weigh risk and benefit ratio.

8.1 Children and adolescents

8.1.1 Diagnostic issues

The diagnosis of bipolar I disorder (BD) in children is challenging and has generated considerable controversy. The major reason for this controversy has to do with the fact that children who present with chronic irritability and/or severe mood dysregulation are often diagnosed with BD in some centres in the US and this has resulted in an increase in apparent rates of BD. A significant proportion of these children also meet criteria for Attention Deficit Hyperactivity Disorder (ADHD) and Oppositional Defiant Disorder (ODD) which makes the diagnosis of BD challenging. Further, classic bipolar symptoms with clear onset and offset are uncommon in children and many of the symptoms of bipolar disorder in children overlap significantly with those of other disorders such as ADHD and ODD. As well, given that cognitive immaturity, mood lability, silliness, and inflated self esteem are not uncommon in younger children, it is understandable these symptoms may sometimes be confused with those of mania such as grandiosity and elation.

8.1.2 Assessment

This should include careful review of current and past symptoms, developmental history, and assessment of current and past functioning. The assessment should include an interview with the child and the parents/caregivers separately and together, and attempts must be made to resolve any inconsistencies in information between the child and parents. Information from teachers is often helpful. When symptoms of euphoria, irritability and grandiosity represent a clear change from baseline functioning, it is easier to make a diagnosis of BD as these children meet the DSM-IV criteria. In children who present with chronic irritability, hyperactivity and severe mood dysregulation, prospective follow up using mood charting and careful documentation of symptom onset and offset is necessary before making a firm diagnosis of BD. Treatment of co-morbid conditions such as ADHD and documentation of manic symptoms in the absence of ADHD would aid in the diagnosis. Prospective follow up data suggest that some of these children do eventually meet DSM-IV criteria for BD.

8.1.3 Differential diagnosis

Chronic irritability, hyperactivity and mood dysregulation are often present in children and adolescents with ADHD, Asperger's syndrome, primary substance abuse, and in those with borderline personality traits/disorder, and hence these must be considered in the differential diagnosis. The features listed in Tables 8.1–8.3 may be helpful in differentiating BD from other conditions.

8.1.4 Treatment options

8.1.4.1 *Lithium*

Although lithium has been used for many years to treat bipolar disorder in children and adolescents, a recent double blind trial in this population failed to show superiority of lithium over placebo. This may be because many children with severe mood dysregulation were included in this trial and it is possible as in adults that lithium is more effective for those with classical bipolar disorder. Adverse events to lithium are more common in younger than older children and lethality of lithium overdose in this population should not be underestimated. Serum levels should rarely exceed 1 mmol/L as higher levels are associated with greater incidence of side effects and poor adherence.

8.1.4.2 *Valproate and other anticonvulsants*

Valproate was effective in one of the two double blind placebo controlled monotherapy trials for acute mania while oxcarbazepine and topiramate are ineffective. Andronization and polycystic ovary syndrome are significant concerns in younger females with valproate.

Carbamazepine and lamotrigine have not been tested in controlled trials in children and adolescents with BD.

Table 8.1 Differential diagnosis of bipolar disorder and ADHD

	Bipolar Disorder	ADHD
Age of onset	Uncommon before age 12	Onset before age 4
Frequency	Episodic	Continuous
Family history	Mood disorders	Disruptive disorders
Clinical Features		
–Grandiosity	Present	Bragging but no grandiosity
–Sleep	Decreased need for sleep	Initial insomnia
–Sexuality	Increased sex drive	Inappropriate sexuality
Response to stimulants	None	Positive
Response to mood stabilizers	Positive	Variable or none

Table 8.2 Differentiating bipolar disorder and primary substance abuse (PSA)

	Bipolar disorder	PSA
Substance	Cocaine or other	Polysubstance
Frequency	Episodic	Continuous
Use related to	Mood problems	Anxiety or disruptive behavioural disorders
Hypo/mania	Present	Absent
Family history	Bipolar or mood disorders	Externalizing or anxiety disorders

Table 8.3 Differentiating bipolar disorder and borderline personality disorder (BPD)

	Bipolar disorder	BPD
Age of onset	May start before puberty	After puberty
Mood dysregulation	Biphasic	In depressive spectrum
Symptoms meet criteria for MDD	Yes	Often do not
During euthymic periods	Reasonable functioning	Dysfunction persists
Family history	Bipolar disorder	Deprivation and abuse
MDD, major depressive disorder.		

8.1.4.3 *Atypical antipsychotics*

Risperidone, quetiapine, aripiprazole, and ziprasidone (not yet approved in UK) were tested in BD children ≥ 10 years and all are effective for acute mania with higher doses yielding more side effects. Response rates were on average 20% to 40% greater with an atypical antipsychotic relative to placebo with an NNT of 3 to 5. Olanzapine was assessed in adolescents with BD with similar response rates. Quetiapine alone or in combination with valproate was more effective than valproate alone for acute mania. Weight gain is a significant concern with atypical antipsychotics in this population although this does not appear to be a major issue with aripiprazole and ziprasidone.

8.1.4.4 *Antidepressants*

No controlled trials assessed the efficacy or safety of antidepressants in children and adolescents with BD. The use of antidepressants in younger population to treat major depression has sparked a lot of controversy with some meta-analyses showing increased risk of suicidal tendencies without any significant apparent benefit in improving major depression. In the absences of any data, great caution must be exercised in using antidepressants in younger subjects with BD and must always be combined with a mood stabilizer.

8.2 Elderly

8.2.1 Clinical presentation and diagnostic issues

First episode mania is uncommon in old age and is often associated with vascular or other brain changes. In those patients who have not had a history of recurrent depressive episodes, an assessment to rule out medical or neurological causes for mania should be undertaken. In the elderly with bipolar disorder, psychotic symptoms are less common in mania but more common in depression compared with younger subjects with bipolar disorder. There is controversy about whether late onset bipolar disorder has higher recurrence rate and longer duration of episodes. Medical co-morbidity is common in elderly with bipolar disorder. About half of the elderly with BD exhibit neurocognitive deficits during euthymia.

8.2.2 Treatment options

There are no large scale placebo controlled trials that specifically assessed treatment of bipolar disorder in the elderly but post-hoc analysis of studies that included elderly BD patients have been conducted.

8.2.2.1 *Acute mania*

Lithium, valproate, and atypical antipsychotics appear to be effective for acute mania. Lithium is particularly effective for those with classical mania and minimal neurological impairment. However, elderly often take other medications or have other medical conditions that may interfere with lithium clearance. Further, elderly may be more sensitive to side effects of lithium. The clearance of valproate is also reduced in the elderly and drugs such as aspirin and warfarin that bind to proteins may increase free fraction of valproate and increase the likelihood of toxicity. As to the atypical antipsychotics, there is a black box warning of increased risk of death in the elderly based on the studies of dementia related psychosis but also the risk of weight gain and metabolic syndrome and the consequent effects on increased cardiovascular morbidity must be considered in the elderly.

8.2.2.2 *Bipolar depression*
In the absence of controlled data in the elderly, bipolar depression in the elderly is managed using the same treatment options as in the adults. However, clinicians must adjust doses taking into consideration pharmacokinetic and pharmacodynamic issues as well as medical co-morbidity in the elderly.

8.2.2.3 *Maintenance treatment*
Post-hoc analysis of trials that included elderly bipolar patients suggest that lamotrigine is effective in preventing mood episodes while lithium was effective in preventing mania in the elderly. Other agents have not been systematically assessed but as in adults, valproate, olanzapine, quetiapine, risperidone, aripiprazole and adjunctive ziprasidone are likely effective.

8.3 Bipolar disorder in women

8.3.1 Clinical issues
Mixed episodes, dysphoric states, depressive episodes, rapid cycling as well as medical comorbidities such as hypothyroidism, obesity and migraine are more common in women than in men. Alcoholism and substance abuse are more common in BD women than in BD men relative to their counterparts in the general population.

8.3.2 Pregnancy counseling
Women with bipolar disorder should be counseled early in the course of the disorder about the potential interactions between psychotropic medications and oral contraceptives and the need for planned pregnancy should they decide to have children (see Table 8.4). When possible a written document explaining the risks and benefits of psychotropic medication vs risks of recurrence of disorder and its consequences and the agreed management options should be signed by the patient and the physician. The decision to continue vs discontinue mood stabilizing medication while a patient is trying to conceive should be made on a case by case basis after carefully

Table 8.4 Counseling for pregnancy planning

Counselling for all women of child-bearing age	Document birth control method Discuss risks of medication exposure during pregnancy Enquire about pregnancy plans Emphasize need for pre-pregnancy consultation
Birth control	Discuss effects of medications on oral contraceptive efficacy Carbamazepine and topiramate decrease levels of OCs OCs decrease lamotrigine levels by 49% and lamotrigine could potentially decrease contraceptive efficacy No known OC interactions with divalproex (semisodium valproate (Depakote®) in the UK), lithium, gabapentin or atypical psychotics
Pre-pregnancy counselling	Provide prenatal counselling at least 3 months before pregnancy Discuss risks of medications during pregnancy, risk to child and mother of antenatal recurrences, and genetic transmission Develop management plans including treatment of recurrence during and after pregnancy Consider a pregnancy contract
Medication use	Prior to conception, consider that conventional antipsychotics and risperidone increase prolactin and may decrease fertility Stable patients may be able to discontinue one or more medications before attempting to conceive and during 1st trimester Assess response to gradual pregravid tapering of medication If medication is required, use monotherapy at minimally effective doses, if possible Assess patient's risk of recurrence and avoid medication during pregnancy especially during first trimester, if possible

considering the risks and benefits of such strategy. Those with a history of severe episodes or multiple recurrent episodes or self harm during episodes may be advised to continue prophylactic medication but the final decision will have to be made by the patient and her partner.

8.3.3 Risks of recurrence during pregnancy

Pregnancy is not protective against episode recurrence. Recurrence rates are 70% during pregnancy. The risk of recurrence is two fold higher and the median time to onset of first recurrence is four fold shorter in women who discontinued vs those continued a mood stabilizer. Most recurrences are depressive or mixed and about half of the recurrences occur during the first trimester.

8.3.4 Management of acute episodes during pregnancy

Lithium, valproate, carbamazepine, and paroxetine have positive evidence for teratogenic risk and should be avoided during the first trimester. The major concerns with lithium are cardiac anomalies and the risk is between 1.2 to 7.7%. Of these, Ebstein Anamoly is the most serious but the absolute risk of this is very low (1 in 1,000 cases). Risk of neural tube defects is a concern with valproate and carbamazepine and it is dose related with valproate and can occur in up to 6% of cases. Lamotrigine is relatively safe although more recent data suggest an association with cleft lip/palate. The data are limited for atypical antipsychotics and they are all rated as category C (risk can not be ruled out) by the FDA. All modern antidepressants also have a rating of C with the exception of bupropion and paroxetine. Bupropion has a rating of B (no evidence of risk in humans) and is preferred during pregnancy while paroxetine should be avoided as it is associated with cardiac anamolies (see Table 8.5). Benzodiazepines should also be avoided during the first 10 weeks of pregnancy because of risk of cleft lip/cleft palate.

If a recurrence occurs during the first trimester, it should be managed with psychosocial approaches when possible. If the risks of not treating outweigh the risks of teratogenic risk, then electroconvulsive therapy or pharmacotherapy should be used to treat the mood episode. The choice of treatment for each phase is dictated by the teratogenic potential of the medications. For instance, for acute mania, atypical antipsychotics are preferable during the first trimester as they have a category C rating in terms of risk. Electroconvulsive therapy (ECT) or quetiapine might be preferable for acute bipolar depression. Antidepressants such as bupropion or an SSRI (except paroxetine) might also be appropriate but these may need to be combined with an atypical antipsychotic to minimize risk of manic switch. Because of changes in fluid volume associated with pregnancy, medication doses may need to be increased during second trimester and early part of third trimester to maintain adequate serum levels and efficacy. The doses may need to be reduced a few days prior to delivery to avoid toxicity. The medication exposure during second and third trimester may be associated with intrauterine fetal death, growth retardation, and neonatal toxicity and patients must be made aware of these risks. Further, exposure to valproate during pregnancy has been reported to be associated with low verbal IQ in children.

8.3.5 Postpartum period

The risk of post-partum mood episodes in women with a history of bipolar disorder is 50% and is almost 70% in those with a history of previous post-partum episodes. Post-partum psychosis occurs in

Table 8.5 Psychotropic medication: teratogenecity and breast feeding risks

Medication	Pregnancy risk	Lactation risk
Lithium	D	L4
Valproate	D	L2
Carbamazepine	D	L2
Lamotrigine	C	L3
Olanzapine	C	L2
Risperidone	C	L3
Quetiapine	C	L4
Aripiprazole	C	L3
Ziprasidone (not yet approved in UK)	C	L4
Haloperidol	C	L2
Bupropion	B	L3
Paroxetine	D	L2
SSRI's except Paroxetine	C	L2 or L3

Pregnancy Risk FDA categories: A= controlled studies show no risk; B= no evidence of risk in humans; C= risk cannot be ruled out; D= positive evidence of risk; X= contraindicated in pregnancy. Lactation risk categories: L1= safest; L2= safer; L3= moderately safe; L4= possibly hazardous; L5= contraindicated.

All psychotropics may carry some risk; physicians should check for current information and weigh the risk/benefit ratio before prescribing these for pregnant or lactating women.

10–20% of deliveries and is associated with a high risk for suicide and infanticide and hence requires urgent medical attention. Prophylaxis with mood stabilizers reduces risk of post-partum mood episodes.

Although concentrations vary, most medications used for treatment of bipolar disorder are secreted in breast milk. Hence, measurement of serum concentrations in infants is not necessary but the infants should be monitored closely for any signs of medication toxicity. Breast feeding should be done before the medication is taken each day to minimize the risk of exposure. Lithium is considered not compatible with breast feeding but valproate and many antidepressants are acceptable (see Table 8.5).

References and further reading

American College of Obstetricians and Gynecologists Committee on Practice Bulletins-Obstetrics. (2008). ACOG Practice Bulletin: Clinical management guidelines for obstetrician-gynecologists number 92, April 2008. Use of psychiatric medications during pregnancy and lactation. *Obstetrics and Gynecology*, **111**(4), 1001–20.

Birmaher B, Axelson D, Monk K et al. (2009). Lifetime psychiatric disorders in school-aged offspring of parents with bipolar disorder: the Pittsburgh Bipolar Offspring study. Arch Gen Psychiatry, 66(3), 287–96.

Carlson GA (2007). Who are the children with severe mood dysregulation, a.k.a. 'rages'? Am J Psychiatry, 164(8), 1140–2.

Krauthammer C, Klerman GL. (1978). Secondary Mania: manic syndromes associated with antecedent physical illness or drugs. Arch Gen Psychiatry, 35(11), 1333–9.

Nulman I, Izmaylov Y, Staroselsky A et al. (2007). 'Teratogenic drugs and chemicals in humans'. In Medication Safety in Pregnancy and Breastfeeding. Ed Gideon Koren. McGraw Hill. Chapter 4 pp. 21–30.

Viguera AC, Cohen LS, Bouffard S et al. (2002). Reproductive decisions by women with bipolar disorder after pre-pregnancy psychiatric consultation. American Journal of Psychiatry, 159(12), 2102–4.

Viguera AC, Newport DJ, Ritchie J et al. (2007). Lithium in breast milk and nursing infants: Clinical implications. Am J Psychiatry, 164(2), 342–5.

Viguera AC, Whitfield T, Baldessarini RJ et al. (2007). Risk of recurrence in women with bipolar disorder during pregnancy: prospective study of mood stabilizer discontinuation. American Journal of Psychiatry, 164(12), 1817–24.

Chapter 9

Patient resources

Key points

- Bipolar disorder often necessitates long-term management. A collaborative approach to management, based on a sound therapeutic relationship, will facilitate engagement and help optimize treatment outcomes
- Patients should be encouraged to take an active role in the management of their own illness and receive psychoeducation about the illness and available treatments options
- There are many facets to managing bipolar disorder and patients are likely to be involved in a range of services by a variety of professionals. Every effort should be made to work cohesively and maintain good communication across all parties
- Patients should be facilitated to access and utilize available resources including peer-support organisations and online resources.

9.1 Self management, psychoeducation, role, and responsibility for illness, insight

For many, bipolar disorder is a recurring illness that is likely to require long-term management or monitoring. Traditionally, the treating doctor or specialist team overseeing care has been allocated the responsibility to fulfil this role however, it is increasingly recognized that the individual is pivotal in their own management and plays an active role in maintaining their own mental health.

Indeed, there is a strong movement led by consumers that focuses on the unique and individual recovery journey, a process that may include progression through a series of stages ranging from a sense of hopelessness and withdrawal from the illness to achieving empowerment through acceptance, better understanding, hope and personal growth. Many mental health services base their treatment philosophy around promoting a recovery-led approach and aim to foster a sense of active involvement in the patient's own care.

Clinicians can facilitate the recovery process by acknowledging and seeking to understand the patient's experience and response to their illness, and also facilitate the development of an understanding of their illness and available treatment options, along with identifying what they can do to maximise their own functioning and minimize the risk of relapse. In this context psychoeducation for the individual and also their family and close supports plays an important role as does promoting healthy lifestyle choices and regular routines to optimize and maintain mental health. Further, clinicians should work with individuals to facilitate an understanding and recognition of their own relapse signals and to practice self awareness by monitoring moods and behaviour patterns.

The goal is to achieve a truly collaborative approach to managing the illness with the flexibility and recognition that there will be times when the consumer can take a lead role in this process and other times when the illness becomes more acute and external care providers will need to adopt a more assertive approach. This can be a difficult balance and one that fluctuates across the illness course.

9.2 Therapeutic relationship, role of professional carers, psychiatrists, psychologists, mental health team, and family

The therapeutic relationship is crucial to effective management of the illness and underpins every facet of treatment. The therapeutic relationship begins at the first point of contact and continues to evolve thereafter. The very nature of bipolar illness means it can involve periods of marked instability and a chaotic lifestyle. Further, pharmacological treatments are not always well tolerated or well-liked by the individual and insight may be limited. Each of these factors contributes to increase the risk of periods of nonadherence to treatment. A therapeutic relationship that is built upon trust, collaboration and openness can improve the likelihood of maintaining engagement in treatment and therefore reduce risk of relapse during these unsettled periods.

The treating team providing care for the person with bipolar disorder can vary depending on the individual, severity of the illness and availability and structure of local services. Care may be based in primary care delivered by a GP or as part of a specialist mental health team, delivered privately or publicly. Typically, public mental health care is provided by a team, led by a psychiatrist but with each patient allocated to a primary care coordinator or case manager who oversees the delivery of care and who has an active role in the day-to-day involvement. This is often a nurse or allied health worker.

Privately, a psychiatrist may be more directly involved in routine monitoring and may then engage various other disciplines such as nursing, psychology or social work to undertake specific tasks. Care is primarily provided in the community setting but at times of acute illness an inpatient admission, sometimes involuntary, may be required to stabilize mental state or to manage any associated short-term risks.

Bipolar disorder affects not only mood, but impacts on all aspects of the individual's life. Therefore effective management should consider a broad range of goals and to achieve this, there are a number of health disciplines that possess expertise across different domains. Although a considerable degree of overlap across professions exists, it is likely that a number of disciplines will need to be involved at different stages to deliver tailored aspects of care. In addition to the role of the medical practitioner, nurses have an active role in the delivery and monitoring of medical and physical care and promoting well-being. Psychological treatments are increasingly recognised as beneficial in bipolar disorder, particularly to help prevent relapses and to improve symptoms during acute depressive phases. In bipolar disorder psychologists employ therapies that target interpersonal relationships, family involvement or maintaining structured routines. Social workers have expertise in working with how the individual relates within their own community and particularly work to optimise social inclusion. Occupational therapists are interested in how people engage in meaningful activities, including work and social functioning, both of which can be significantly impacted upon by bipolar disorder.

Bipolar disorder does not affect the individual in isolation and often the family is closely involved and need to be integrated into treatment. The term 'carer' is often used to refer to those family members or friends who are responsible for providing direct support or care to a person with a mental illness. 'Carers', and indeed other close family members, will likely require emotional support, education about the illness and treatment options, practical strategies to manage difficult behaviours or in times of crisis and can provide an active role in helping to monitor mental health.

9.3 Self help groups, consumer associations, and the role of government organizations

Peer-led organizations can provide an important source of emotional and social support as well as educational resources. Some people find particular benefit in obtaining support from others with shared experiences and such groups often promote a consumer-driven recovery-led approach. Availability varies on locality but usually involves a mixture of smaller community-based groups as well as larger national organizations often with accompanying online resources.

Where required, external agencies or organizations may also be involved by providing disability support or assisting with other non-clinical aspects of care, such as vocational support programmes.

9.4 Web-based interventions and resources

The advent of the internet has provided an abundance of resources that are freely available to access about bipolar disorder and related topics. Accessing the internet can be encouraged as part of promoting self-management and patients should be directed to particularly reputable and well-resourced websites. This can be an opportunity for further psychoeducation and patients should be encouraged to discuss with their clinician any questions they have about the information they are reading. There is also an emerging interest in web-based psychological interventions that are likely to play a role in the management of bipolar disorder. These are particularly focused on providing online programmes for structured interventions such as cognitive behavioural therapy.

References and further reading

Berk M, Berk L, and Castle D (2004). A collaborative approach to the treatment alliance in bipolar disorder. *Bipolar Disorders*, **6**(6), 504–18.

Oades L, Deane F, Crowe T, Lambert WG, Kavanagh D, and Lloyd C (2005). Collaborative recovery: an integrative model for working with individuals who experience chronic and recurring mental illness. *Australasian Psychiatry*, **13**(3), 279–84.

Useful online resources

www.bipolarconnect.com   Lists web-based resources for bipolar disorder
www.dbsalliance.org   Depression and bipolar support alliance
www.bphope.com   Online newsletter for people with bipolar disorder

Index

Printed in the USA/Agawam, MA
October 16, 2013

580987.099